STOP!

DON'T KILL ME

Understanding the Impact of
Racism in Healthcare
A Toolkit for Your Survival

Dr. E. J. Johnson

STOP! DON'T KILL ME

Understanding the Impact of Racism in Healthcare. A Toolkit for Your Survival

Walton Publishing House

Houston, Texas

www.waltonpublishinghouse.com

Printed in the United States of America

Library of Congress Cataloging in-Publication Data under herein.
ISBN:
Digital- 978-1-953993-53-3
Paperback- 978-1-953993-54-0

CONTENTS

INTRODUCTION

I thought that I was going to die. It was Tax Day, April 15, 2019, a day that many of us dread. However, my dread was elevated because I was ordered to have an emergency CT scan that was followed by my third visit to the emergency room in four weeks. I was denied once again the life-saving surgery to remove my ruptured appendix. I was told that my pain was not that bad, however, I felt that my body was shutting down. The thoughts that kept racing my head with each emergency room visit were, *"Stop! Don't Kill Me."* The thought of dying from acute appendicitis was not far-fetched. My husband's sister went to the emergency room due to severe abdominal pain. She was diagnosed with acute appendicitis and sent home with antibiotics. Her appendix ruptured and she tragically died.

What we had in common was that we were both Black women and our healthcare emergencies were both summarily dismissed by a racist healthcare system that does not value Black life. I prayed to God that my life would not end and begged for His mercy and guidance. I had already consulted with four surgeons, and all agreed with the first surgeon who had decided to delay my surgery. I needed to urgently find a surgeon willing to listen to me and more importantly, I needed that surgeon to respect my humanity. I needed a surgeon who knew that my life had value.

As I continued my prayer, God directed my path to a surgeon who had performed my husband's colon cancer surgery in 2006. Ironically, I would meet that same surgeon in 2013, as a healthcare consultant. I recounted how I had been in hospitals literally hundreds of times during my career. I had worked on a myriad of healthcare improvement projects that resulted in new processes, procedures, programs, and toolkits that helped to improve healthcare outcomes for thousands of patients and families. I also knew the long tragic history of Black patients being ignored, devalued, and marginalized. I had witnessed it up close during work and now I was experiencing it first-hand. I thank God that I was able to find my voice and took the necessary actions to save my life. My husband's surgeon agreed to perform my appendectomy and I am still here, blessed with a new calling. I realized that I needed to share my knowledge of the racist healthcare system to help save lives.

Whenever I shared my story about my healthcare nightmare with family, friends and, colleagues, all would express three sentiments. The first was to express empathy for what I experienced; the second was to tell me that I was blessed to be alive and the third was to ask me what I was going to do about what happened to me. It was that third response that stuck with me, what *I was going to do? What action would I take*? This is something that I have wrestled with for two years. Finally, it was God who told me to write my book to help Black women, the primary caregivers for their families. God told me to use my "voice" to help others to find their "voices" to address the racist healthcare system. I created the *VOICE Your Concerns for Your Healthcare Toolkit* that not only gives the workflows on how healthcare works, but also gives you a list of questions that you should ask healthcare providers during your healthcare encounters in the emergency room, urgent care center, primary physician office, specialist office, labor and delivery, and operating room. You will also learn what actions to take if your healthcare concerns are not addressed.

It is crucial to address the healthcare equity gap experienced by millions of Black women who are frustrated with a healthcare system that does not always see their humanity. I will share my experiences as a healthcare consultant where I bear witness to how racism impacts healthcare in the same way that it impacts education, employment, and justice. I will also share my experiences as a patient and how through the power of God, I was able to find my voice to take action to save my life. The knowledge shared in this book will help you to navigate the complex healthcare system. As of February 2022, the COVID-19 global pandemic, which began in December 2019, has infected and killed over 75 million Americans and over 900,000 lives respectively.[1] It is shocking that at the start of the pandemic, Black Americans were as high as four times more likely to die of COVID-19 compared to white Americans.[2]

My heart still aches for a dear sister, Dr. Susan Moore, a Black doctor who died of COVID-19 on December 10, 2020. Dr. Moore chronicled her horrific ordeal with a video post on Facebook. In the video, she explains how she was a victim of a racist healthcare system, where white nurses and a white doctor at the hospital in suburban Indianapolis, where she was being treated for COVID-19, had downplayed her complaints of pain. She stated he told her that he felt uncomfortable giving her more narcotics and suggested that she would be discharged. I was in shock to learn that Dr. Moore, a phenomenal Black physician, was told that she would be discharged while still suffering from COVID-19.

In her video, she stated the following:

> "I was crushed. He made me feel like I was a drug addict... I put forth and I maintain if I was white, I wouldn't have to go through that. This is how Black people get killed, when you

> send them home and they don't know how to fight for themselves." [3]

Upon her passing two weeks after her first hospital visit, her son shared the following:

> "Nearly every time she went to the hospital, she had to advocate for herself, fight for something in some way, shape or form, just to get baseline, proper care." [4]

After Dr. Moore passed away, in a December 24, 2020 press release, the CEO of the Indiana University Hospital, Dennis M. Murphy, described Dr. Moore as a complex patient. He then blamed Dr. Moore for the horrific treatment that she endured at his hospital by stating the following:

> "The nursing staff treating her for coronavirus, may have been intimidated by a knowledgeable patient who was using social media to voice her concerns and critique the care that they were delivering." [5]

Dr. Moore is not alone regarding Black women and harrowing healthcare experiences. I am a huge fan of both Venus and Serena Williams. I cried with both pain and joy as my husband and I watched the 2021 movie "King Richard," which chronicles the story of how Richard Williams created a 78-page plan for his daughters, Venus and Serena. The goal was for both of them to become the number one tennis players in the world. Not only did Richard Williams achieve his vision with both of his prodigious daughters achieving the coveted world number one ranking, but it was surpassed with Serena becoming the greatest player of all time, winning twenty-three grand slams! My heart ached as I read the April 5th, 2022, *Elle* magazine published essay authored by Serena Williams, entitled "How Serena Williams Saved Her Own Life." Black women are nearly three times more likely to die after childbirth than white women. Serena Williams was almost one of them. Here, in her own words, she recounts her story. [6] I knew that Serena had almost died after giving birth, but to read her own words only magnified the significant problem with racism in healthcare.

In her riveting essay, Serena shares that after her emergency C-section to deliver her daughter, Olympia on September 1, 2017, she had to fight for her life by voicing her concerns about her healthcare. She writes:

> "In 2010, I learned I had blood clots in my lungs—clots that, had they not been caught in time, could have killed me. Ever since then, I've lived in fear of them returning. It wasn't a one-off; I'm at high risk for blood clots. I asked a nurse, 'When do I start my heparin drip? Shouldn't I be on that now?' The response was, 'Well, we don't really know if that's what you need to be on right now.' No one was really listening to what I was saying." [6]

Unfortunately, Serena had to have a second surgery to close her C-section which had re-opened after a coughing spat due to blood clots. After this surgery, Serena once again had to voice her concerns about her healthcare as noted below:

> "I felt like I was dying. I spoke to the nurse. I told her: 'I need to have a CAT scan of my lungs bilaterally, and then I need to be on my heparin drip.' She said, 'I think all this medicine is making you talk crazy.' I said, 'No, I'm telling you what I need: I need the scan immediately. And I need it to be done

> with dye.' I guess I said the name of the dye wrong, and she told me I just needed to rest. But I persisted: 'I'm telling you, this is what I need.' Finally, the nurse called my doctor, and she listened to me and insisted we check. I fought hard, and I ended up getting the CAT scan." [6]

Serena was insistent and received life-saving surgery. Her following statement is so personal to me:

> "Being heard and appropriately treated was the difference between life or death for me." [6]

Dr. Moore's fatal experience, and Serena Williams' near-death experience both demonstrate what many Black women, albeit professionals in their fields, including myself know to be true in America; education cannot protect you from mistreatment, whether in the hospital, at a bank, at school, or any other institution. You have to find your voice and share your concerns about how you are being treated during a healthcare encounter. Unfortunately, sometimes, your voice may be what is needed to save your life, and perhaps those that you love.

During my healthcare nightmare, I realized the need for Black women to have useful information on how to navigate the complex 18 trillion-dollar American healthcare system. It is also essential to understand the historical context of why, for centuries, Black patients continue to land at the bottom of every negative health outcome metric from birth, with the highest infant mortality rates, to death, with the highest premature death rates in America. I want you to know how sincerely that Black healthcare matters.

The challenge for Black patients is understanding how to navigate the racist healthcare system, to ensure that they do not become one of the disheartening statistics. I believe in the adage that "knowledge is power" and therefore understanding the origins of the American healthcare system is critical. In addition, there is a need to know what to do when you feel that you are not receiving fair and equitable healthcare. The racist lie that Black people do not feel physical or emotional pain is deeply rooted in the dehumanization of our enslaved ancestors. Although physical pain is a primary indicator that something is wrong with the body, the pain of a Black patient is often not taken seriously. Despite the clear medical reality that I was physically suffering from acute appendicitis, I was told that my pain was not that bad and sent home with antibiotics. You must be able to find your voice and speak up against a biased and systematically racist healthcare system to save the lives of you and your family.

PART 1

UNDERSTANDING RACISM IN HEALTHCARE

CHAPTER 1:
HOW I BECAME A HEALTHCARE CONSULTANT

M*om almost died and is still in the hospital"* are words that I will never forget. As a young girl growing up in segregated Pittsburgh, Pennsylvania in the 1960s, I remember that if a family member was ill, the family doctor would come to our home and literally go to the bedside of a loved one. However, my young brain was desperately trying to process what was different this time. My older sister explained to me that the doctor did not come to our home because our mother had to go to the hospital to have a baby. I would learn years later that she nearly died while giving birth to my brother and had stayed in the hospital for over a month. This was still challenging for me to comprehend at the age of six. I just remember me and my sister praying for Mom to come home. I really needed her because I was about to have my first experience at a hospital.

It was a school day morning and I remember that my new baby brother was crying. However, my mother was still in the hospital. My aunt was there helping the family during her absence. She had completed my hair and directed me to the kitchen for breakfast. In the kitchen, my eldest sister, who was twelve years old was preparing our breakfast. The choice was always between grits, oatmeal, or cream of wheat. My mom was an advocate for her children starting the school day with a hot meal. That day, it was my favorite of the three, grits. My sister had placed the hot pot of grits on the table under a potholder and used a ladle to scoop out one small serving per plate.

As she prepared each plate, I noticed that one plate had a double serving. My eyes were wide with excitement as my young brain devised a plan to grab that plate with the extra serving before my older siblings noticed. As I reached for the plate, I was oblivious to my sister still scooping the last serving. Then it happened. My small six-year-old hand was covered with smoldering grits. I screamed in pain. My aunt rushed into the kitchen and removed the hot grits from my hand with a kitchen towel. My next memory is sitting on a hospital bed and this beautiful Black nurse was helping me. I remember how she gently applied some salve on my hand and then wrapped it with white gauze. It was my dominant hand and I remember my dad asking how long the burn would take to heal. He was concerned that I may not be able to do my schoolwork. When I returned home, my eldest sister was in tears as she apologized and assured me that she did not see my small hand. Overall, my first hospital experience was very positive because of my Black nurse and the support of my loving family. This belief was further reinforced with a famous and ground-breaking television show.

In 1968, a new television show aired aptly titled, *Julia* starring Diahann Carroll as a nurse and widowed mother of one son named, Corey. I loved that show because it reminded me of the nurse who became my angel. In retrospect, I realize the importance of having Black healthcare providers. Growing up in a segregated city, allowed me to see how Black neighbors collaborated and supported one another to achieve better opportunities for their children.

At the age of eight, my family moved into a six-bedroom three-story home located in the Black "Homewood" neighborhood. On our one short block, there lived a Black doctor, three Black teachers, a Black funeral home director, a Black singer, and myriad Black entrepreneurs. Needlessly to say, that environment had a profound impact on my life. I was living on the same street as some of my teachers. I even had the opportunity to babysit for some of them. This was absolutely life-changing for me to be enveloped in a sea of so many Black professionals in our close-knit neighborhood including those in healthcare.

Many of the neighborhood Black healthcare professionals worked at the Alma Illery Health Center. The health center was named after Dr. Alma Illery, a civil rights activist, who single-handedly lobbied Congress in 1944 to pass a bill establishing January 5th, as George Washington Carver Day. This was in memory of Tuskegee Institute's famed Black scientist. In addition, Dr. Illery, due to her activism on behalf of the poor was welcomed at the White House during five presidencies.[7] The Alma Illery Health Center was a short walk away from our home. This is the center that my family and I went to for not only our annual check-ups but also our routine medical and dental care. The center was newly constructed in the predominately Black neighborhood of Homewood. Thus, during my childhood, I was exposed to essential Black healthcare professionals, who like my Black teachers at my predominately Black School, treated me and my family with love and care.

My childhood healthcare experiences included the beautiful Black nurse who took excellent care of me after my hand-burning incident. Unfortunately, I was never to experience that feeling of perfect healthcare again. My hand did heal, however, my future encounters with the white controlled healthcare system, have left a wound that is much too deep to heal.

Although I was intrigued by the Black doctors and nurses that I had met as a child, I pondered the possibility of becoming a doctor. However, it was during my high school years, that I knew that I wanted to become a chemical engineer. Why chemical engineering? I absolutely loved chemistry and math during high school. I attended a Black high school with a Black principal and Black teachers. Mrs. Peters and Mrs. James taught algebra and geometry respectively. Mrs. Williams taught chemistry. All were role models of why young Black women needed both classroom lessons and life lessons. However, it was my ultimate role model, my mother, who taught me that with God, all things are possible. She wrote in my autograph book from my 7th-grade graduation, "We expect great things from you." She also told me that one day, I would be on the cover of *Essence* magazine. In addition, my parents, similar to tennis dad, Richard Williams, had a vision. Their vision was that all eight of their children would go to college and graduate. My father would emphasize, "You will not just go to college. Many people go to college. You must also graduate from college."

With encouragement from my teachers and family, I decided to pursue uncharted waters. I matriculated to the University of Pittsburgh to begin my studies in chemical engineering. The Pitt Engineering Impact Program (PEIP) was a so-called "Minority Engineering Program" (MEP) that began in 1969 to help increase the number of Black engineers across the United States as described below:[8]

> "In 1969 the late Dr. Karl Lewis (1/15/1936-3/5/2019) founded the IMPACT Program at the University of Pittsburgh to encourage minority and financially and culturally disadvantaged students to enter and graduate from the field of engineering. The six-week program prepared incoming first year students through exposure to university academic life, development of study skills, academic and career

counseling, and coursework to reinforce strengths or remedy weaknesses. Many Pitt alumni today still note the role that Lewis and IMPACT had on their personal and professional lives."[8]

As an alumnus of the Impact Program, it undoubtedly served as an important bridge program to assist with my transition from a Black high school and neighborhood to a predominately white university. Ironically, in 1979, the University of Pittsburgh had its highest rate of Black enrollment since it began admitting Black students as shown in Figure 1.[9] Apparently, this was in response to years of protest that culminated with a sit-in at the historic Cathedral of Learning. It was a struggle as I yearned for my supportive Black teachers who celebrated my curiosity and passion for excellence compared to the white university professors who seemed enraged that I dared to take a seat in their classroom. I felt that as one of the few Black engineering students, I was seen as new prey for them to taunt and tease relentlessly.

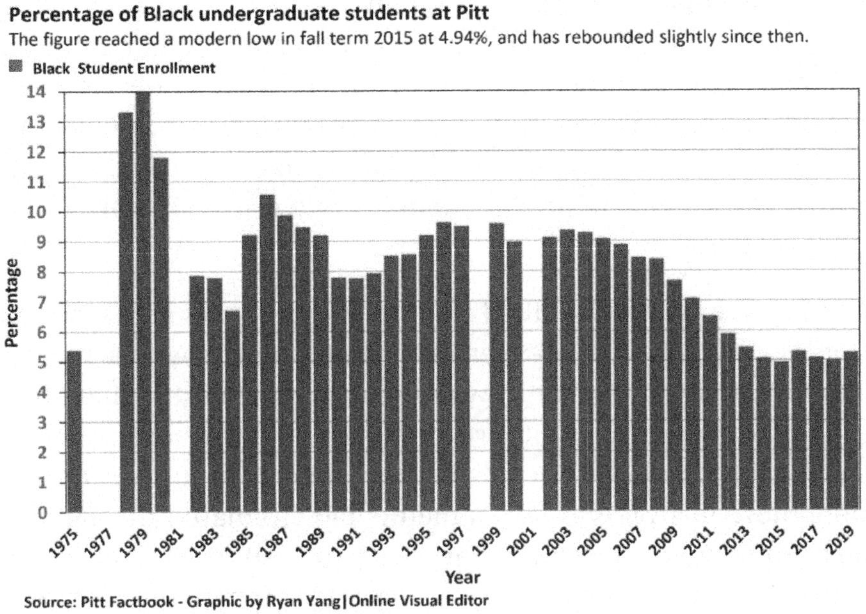

Figure 1 University of Pittsburgh Black Undergraduate Enrollment 1975 to 2019

It was my freshman year, and I had my first engineering course taught by Professor Coleman, a thin man with glasses, who wore the same green suit at every lecture. There were approximately two hundred students in the large lecture hall with stadium seating and electronic whiteboards. He used a microphone to ensure that all students could hear his shrill voice. As one of only two Black students in the class, I sat at a two-person desk in the front of the hall. You could only imagine my surprise that day when I heard my name called by the professor for me to stay after class. The professor knew me because I always asked myriad questions, to which he often responded with disdain. He wanted to let me know that I scored a 94 out of 100 on the first exam and wanted to understand how was I able to accomplish, to him, what was a most "remarkable" feat. He asked me the following: Did my parents go to college? What high school did I attend?

How many children were in my family? Were they all as smart as me? I remembered responding that I was one of eight children and that I was the dumbest of them all. The look on his face was priceless. It was a combination of surprise, fear, and finally anger. I was not the anomaly that he had expected. There were at least seven other potential students who were even more intelligent than me.

My freshman year was filled with those moments in which the professors all tried to desperately understand how I achieved high marks. Again, to them, I was a strange enigma and there had to be a reason why I outperformed the majority of my white peers. I had made the Dean's list throughout that year. By my sophomore year, it was as if a memo had circulated throughout the campus with a warning that each professor must ensure my failure by any means necessary. My freshman exams were mostly multiple choice with unequivocal right or wrong answers. This was quite different during subsequent years in which my engineering exams were subjectively graded. Although I could derive the correct answer, the methodology could be challenged, and the professor could arbitrarily lower my final grade. It became a war with my professors as I challenged their biased grading methods. Despite my countless obstacles, I graduated from the university earning my Bachelor of Science in chemical engineering in 1983 with honors.

My next step was to begin my chemical engineering career at a major corporation and earn a living. However, in 1983, Ronald Reagan was the president, and the Black American unemployment rate was 19.5 % compared to 8.4% for white Americans.[10] At the time of graduation, I recall that less than 10% of the chemical engineering graduates had jobs in their fields. Therefore, like many others, I stayed at the university and went directly to graduate school. There were only 30 graduate students in my class compared to the 121 students that graduated from the undergraduate program. There was one other Black student, Victor

Rodgers in the chemical engineering master's degree program. Victor and his identical twin brother, Vincent made history as the first Black professors in chemical engineering and physics at the University of Iowa. They were both featured in *Jet* magazine in 1993.[11] Needless to say, Victor became my source of emotional support and sanity while trying to navigate an engineering institution that was more sexist than racist.

During my first semester of graduate school, I quickly found out that sexism, in addition, to racism would be my new hurdle. My graduate thermodynamics course required a group project. Unfortunately, I was denied entry to any of the five groups. When I explained my dilemma to the professor, he assigned me to a team comprised of five male foreign students. I thought to myself, this is so unfair. The groups should have been assigned randomly; however, I was determined to make it work. During our first group meeting, I remember being told that I could type the final report. I refused to be belittled and boldly declared that we all would share equally on aspects of the project. I became fast friends with Kim Chong because one of my Black male friends was also named Kim, I thought that it was ironic that I would meet another male named Kim. I endured several pranks throughout the project, including the constant changing of the computer password preventing me access to the project files. I would constantly have to get the new password from Kim. I was determined to make sure that our project was successful.

Then the worst happened. At the end of the project, in which I worked twice as hard as my male team members, they received "A's" and I received a "B" on the same project. When I asked, "Why?" The professor stated that he did not believe that as the only woman on the team, I actually worked as hard as the men. I was livid. That was it for me. I was both physically and mentally exhausted. I took my grievance to the only Black professor in the chemical engineering department. I needed some sage advice. Dr. Alfred Bishop was a brilliant professor and my mentor and recommended that I file a complaint for both racism and sexism with Student Affairs. Despite their investigation, I received a very limp apology, however, my project grade was unchanged.

That experience helped to reinforce my reality that engineering was definitely more sexist than it was racist. I chose to leave the university and enter the workforce. My strategy was that I would at least get paid for the discrimination that I would face throughout life. In 1984, I was one of the three Black women engineers to join the Westinghouse Nuclear Engineering Department. We were pioneers and steadfast to leave our mark in nuclear engineering. I even became an ambassador for nuclear engineering, doing TV shows, radio, and tours to high schools sharing the importance of "clean" nuclear energy juxtaposed to "dirty" energy derived from coal. I was doing well in the industry and completed my master's degree part-time in 1987. It was then that I decided to get my doctorate. In 1997, I made history, as the first Black person (man or woman) to earn a Ph.D. in chemical engineering from the University of Pittsburgh. In 2004, after working for many years, I earned my MBA to hone the requisite skills for my part-time consulting business with the goal to parlay it into a full-time endeavor.

In 2001, I was able to launch my company, Pioneer Training & Consulting which focused on continuous improvement utilizing basic engineering principles. As an engineer, my job is to identify, assess, measure, and analyze a problem and then provide sustainable solutions. As an engineering consultant, I was able to secure a role at an international pharmaceutical company. The company was based in Sweden with locations around the world including the United States and the United Kingdom. I later became the first Learning & Development Manager of the Operations Strategy & Capability department responsible for the continuous learning of over fifteen hundred U.S-based employees. I created a three-year strategy focused on both behavioral and technical competencies. I was able to identify adult learning theories that included emotional intelligence, intra-cultural competency, and diversity training. In my role as the Global Medical Science Manager, I was responsible for creating a Global Physician Leadership Program and a Global Standard Operating Procedure (SOP) training program. It was during my years of creating global training programs for physicians, and scientists that I was able to understand the importance of having respect for cultural diversity and inclusion. I was also a project manager for a Clinical Pharmacology Unit (CPU) which is where new drugs are tested on healthy patients for safety and efficacy prior to the clinical trial with patients who have the disease. This was performed globally.

As the global director for the Quality Management Continuous Improvement Department with team members in Sweden, the United Kingdom, and the United States, one of the key projects was the creation of a new Clinical Development Quality Framework. My team was responsible for developing new processes that would improve clinical development efficiency. Once the processes were improved, I created new Standard Operating Procedures (SOPs) and aligned all relevant information technology platforms. The new system enabled anyone to track all stages of the clinical development system. For example, once the clinical trial was launched, the trial data is collected and ultimately submitted to both the FDA and EU participants for drug approval. The goal was to reduce the time to develop a new drug from twelve years to eight years.

During my ten years in the pharmaceutical business sector, as both a consultant and a quality improvement expert, I was able to transfer my quality management and clinical development skills to healthcare delivery science. By 2010, more engineers were working in hospitals, emergency rooms, operating rooms, and medical offices to improve efficiency and reduce costs. In fact, the applications of manufacturing lean principles for problem-solving had gained acceptance in healthcare. The fact that I was an engineer with an MBA and a Lean Six Sigma Master Black Belt (process improvement expert) made me uniquely qualified as a healthcare delivery consultant.

CHAPTER 2: THE U.S. HEALTHCARE SYSTEM – WHAT YOU NEED TO KNOW

Inside Look Into The Healthcare System

The problem with healthcare delivery was the ability to assess systems to identify their value. Why was this important? In 2010, the new Affordable Care Act (ACA), required that the healthcare systems change from fee-for-service to value-based care. This had a dramatic effect on hospital systems and medical office practices. The objective was to reduce the need for hospitalization by providing preventative care including screening programs. For example, in a fee-for-service model, each time a poorly treated diabetes patient goes to an emergency room, the hospital is reimbursed for each visit. Thus, the hospital benefits from patients that do not receive proper care because proper care would reduce emergency room visits. In a value-based outcome care model (see figure 2), it is crucial for the healthcare provider, the primary care physician, to actually treat the diabetic patient and not be paid for excessive emergency room utilization.

The Value-Based Payment Model has a theoretical definition for the value equation:

Value = (Quality + Service)/ Cost

The healthcare value equation is a function of healthcare quality, healthcare service, and healthcare cost. Each variable should be measurable, however, only service and cost have defined metrics. The service is measured by both performance outcomes, clinical outcomes, and patient experience. The cost is measured by both direct patient costs and indirect patient costs. However, there are no metrics for quality.

The quality of a product is very much different from the quality of service. As a customer, if you purchase a product, for example, a pair of pants for a child, however, when you arrive home, and your child tries the pants on, the zipper is defective. You then return to the store to return the item. The quality of service would be assessed by how well you were treated during the return process. Did the store clerk treat you with respect and provide helpful information to aid in your decision-making? Did you exchange the pants for the same or different product, or did you obtain a refund?

It is important for a theoretical quality healthcare delivery model to be a function of the knowledge of the people engaged in the patient encounter: the provider, patient, and patient advocate. The patient advocate can be family, friends, or a paid healthcare advocate. This theoretical quality model must also address the racial bias both explicit and implicit.

The theoretical quality equation is as follows:

$$Quality = \frac{(\text{Provider Knowledge} + \text{Patient Knowledge} + \text{Patient Advocate Knowledge})}{\text{Racial Bias Factor}}$$

The medical profession continues to evolve with new evidenced-based practices becoming more important to patient outcomes. If a provider does not have current knowledge of the illness or disease, the quality would be reduced. Likewise, if the patient does not share all their knowledge about what is happening to their body, the quality will be reduced. For example, Paul is doing home repairs and falls off a ladder. His wife, Angie, drives him to the emergency room. During the consult, Paul explains the event to the emergency room physician and states that he injured his knee and hand during the fall. However, he does not mention that he hit his head on the floor. This omission can reduce the quality of healthcare delivery. However, his wife Angie witnessed the event and describes how his head hit the floor, thereby improving the quality. Angie provided additional knowledge as a healthcare advocate.

The final variable is the *Racial Bias Factor* which can be rated as high, medium, or low. A rating of high would be assigned to explicit racial bias. For example, a Black patient arrives in the emergency room and complains of excruciating abdominal pain. The emergency room physician has been trained that Black people have a higher pain tolerance than white people and does not assess the pain properly. This explicit racial bias can have a highly negative impact on quality. On the low end, implicit bias can also reduce the quality of healthcare service. For example, a nurse is aware of a new yoga program for all cancer patients, however, she does not think that her Black patients would be interested, thus she does not share the program with her patients. The quality is reduced because the nurse withholds important healthcare due to racial bias.

My transition from a chemical engineer and then a pharmaceutical executive to a healthcare consultant was, more than eye-opening. I was not surprised by the racism that I encountered in healthcare. I was quickly reminded of Dr. Martin Luther King, who surmised racism as the controlling of institutions that discriminate on the basis of color or ethnicity. [12] Thus, institutional systemic racism has wreaked havoc in the Black community and is based on centuries of discriminatory practices.

However, what is sad is that some members of the Black community, having suffered over 400 years of institutional racism, will defend white supremacy racism, and accuse the person reporting the racism as being the actual racist. To me, this would be akin to accusing a rape victim of being a rapist. Both the rapist and racist must have power and control to enact their dastardly deeds.

The best-selling *White Fragility* author, Robin DiAngelo, challenges white people to rethink how they define racism. She states the following:

> "Racism's survival doesn't depend on our agreement or beliefs — even if you don't think people should be treated differently because of their race, they automatically will be mistreated across those systems: education, health care, criminal justice, housing, banking, economics, language, technology, media representation, ideology and so on. If we don't interrupt the systems we live within, then we're complicit."[13]

Thus, these key systems: education, healthcare, criminal justice, housing, banking, economics, language, technology, media representation, and are controlled by institutional racism.

In reading *White Fragility*, I can't help but wonder if the author read *The Isis Papers: The Keys to the Colors* by critically acclaimed Howard University professor and psychiatrist, Dr. Francis Cress Welsing. In her 1991 book, she shares that white supremacy racism controls nine areas of people's activities:

> "The Cress Theory was based upon the insightful work of Neely Fuller Jr., author of The United Independent Compensatory Code/System/ Concept - a textbook/workbook for thought, speech and/or action for victims of racism (White supremacy). Fuller, the founder of the racism/counter· racism concept, was the very first victim of racism to understand it as a global system of organized behavior (thought, speech and action) for white supremacy domination in all areas of people activity (economics, education, entertainment, labor, law, politics, religion, sex and war). In other words, he recognized that all activity and behavior encompassed by the white supremacy system had and has its origin in the dynamic of racism. Additionally, Fuller understood that racism contained the seeds and origin of counter-racism, the behavior dynamic of liberation for the non-white victims of white supremacy. His work led me to question the necessity of the global White collective to evolve such a system of unjust behavior. The result was The Cress Theory of Color Confrontation and Racism (White Supremacy)." [14]

Ironically, Dr. Frances Cress Welsing recognized the importance of adding a tenth activity in her later writings called "Health." The history of racism in healthcare will be explored in depth in future chapters. However, before the exploration, we must understand why does white supremacy racism continue in America?

The simple truth is that white supremacy racism works well in America. Let's simply examine the origins of racism: a group of white men, or should I dare say, white scholarly men, created a social construct to justify the oppression, suppression, and marginalization of human beings literally across the globe. It is important for the system to have a visual management system to make it easy to control. The hue of a person or "hue-man" could be delineated into four colored categories, White, Yellow, Red, and Black. Thereby, the racial caste system in America was created and still exists today with a lot more hues due to hundreds of years of rape and miscegenation.

It is also important to understand the etymology of the word "race." It is a homograph: a word that is spelled the same and pronounced the same but has different meanings. In the *Britannica* dictionary, the noun, races, has two definitions. The first definition is "a contest or competition in which different people try to do something first."[15] The second definition for the word race is "one of the groups that people can be divided into based on certain physical qualities such as skin color."[15] For me, it is intended that this made-up social construct with no biological foundation is called "race" because the quality of life that you experience is a competition. A competition in which white people have advantages and always win. How? In this faux competition, white people have the power and control of major institutions including the government, hospitals, pharmaceutical companies, and insurance companies.

In healthcare, racial health disparities have been measured and reported annually for decades. The results are consistently the same year to year. White people are "winning" with better healthcare outcomes compared to Black people and other racial minorities. This should not be a surprise since the system was created to address white illness and disease, and not the healthcare needs of Black citizens In America, each aspect of healthcare service delivery is controlled by white people from the hospital CEOs to government policymakers.

In 1923, there were nearly 200 Black hospitals in America that served millions of Black families There are only four Black hospitals today.[16] In 1940, only 2.7% of all physicians in America were Black men in comparison, in 2018, only 2.6% of all physicians were Black men. In 1900, 1940, and 2020, the percentage of all Black physicians in the United States, was 1.3%, 2.8%, and 5.8 % respectively.[17] The unvarnished truth is that not much has changed in healthcare during the last 120 years despite the known research that Black patients who have Black doctors have significantly better clinical outcomes and closing of the health disparity gaps. The healthcare system, similar to the educational system, has a structure that is deeply rooted in discriminatory practices in which Black consumers have no power in decision-making. However, as a healthcare consultant for ten years, I was able to bear witness to a system that not only killed thousands of patients each year due to medical negligence but was intentionally complex to mask accountability.

Working in the pharmaceutical industry for ten years, I learned about the structure of clinical trials and how trial data is obtained and analyzed. The healthcare measurement systems that are used to define what is normal are historically based on white bodies and usually male. For new drugs, the majority of clinical trials in America usually have white male participants. Why? This is because women in childbearing years may get pregnant, and the pharmaceutical company fears that a new drug could harm the unborn fetus. Keep in mind, that whenever you take a new medication for the very first time, that is your clinical trial. If you have a headache, and you take an over-the-counter (OTC) pain medication for the first time, you have no idea if that medication will work for you and your body. The clinical trial was based on white men and their physiology, their metabolism, and more importantly their response to whether the new pain medication was effective. However, we have blind faith and trust that the new medication will work at the dose prescribed. Working in healthcare delivery for a decade, I learned that finding the right medication type and dosage for any disease is based on trial and error. For example, a person who just had open heart surgery will be given strong narcotics to relieve pain, however, each patient will respond differently, and the dosage will be modified to meet the needs of that specific patient. These decisions to order pharmaceutical drugs are made by primarily white physicians.

Interestedly, in the pharmaceutical industry, all employees received ethical training that stressed patient safety and the ramifications for both the company and individuals. Unlike, the healthcare system, in which clearly the system was stressed as the responsible party instead of the actions of a specific individual. When I began working on a new project, I would immediately request all of the current standard operating procedures (SOPs) for the processes. In both the chemical and pharmaceutical industries, I reviewed, updated, and created SOPs. Instead of SOPs, I was often presented with policies and guidelines. So, what is the big deal? The difference for me is huge because when I author a new SOP, it states a very standardized way to get work done and ensures that the product or service is produced the same way each time without deviation. I see policies and guidelines as more of a recommendation of what should occur and allow more opportunity for deviations. My role as consultant enabled me to lead projects that resulted in the development of much-needed standardized work in the form of clinical pathways, standardized care plans, and standardized operating procedures for many healthcare institutions.

In October 2019, I received the National Oncology Journal Clinical Pathway of the Year Award for leading a team to address cancer care in a standardized way. It is imperative to create standardized care to address health disparities that lead to unequal care experiences and clinical outcomes. It is well known that Black patients are often the recipient of poorer healthcare delivery. The novel clinical pathway addressed cancer patients receiving both chemotherapy and radiation treatments with an exceptionally high risk for hospital admission due to pain management and lack of control of their diabetes or COPD. This higher utilization of emergency room visits yielded more hospital admissions and 30-day readmissions.

I also led a multidisciplinary team that included the emergency department physicians to address why cancer patients are admitted to the hospital at a higher rate unnecessarily. This results in higher costs without the benefit of better clinical outcomes. In some cases, the hospital admission can be extremely disruptive to scheduled chemical therapy or radiation therapy appointments. The clinical pathway created a clear structured process with activities by role, i.e., nurse, physician, oncologist, nurse navigator, etc. to ensure that all patients received the same care. In addition, the nurse navigators used a software platform that monitored their care delivery by task. A nurse navigator is seen as the "conductor" of the patient's healthcare team and coordinates all appointments with the doctors, social workers, speech therapists, specialists, dieticians, and psychologists.

One of the key challenges for cancer patients is that their nurse navigator must complete all assigned tasks on time. For example, if the patient had a hospital admission, ideally the nurse navigator should follow up with the patient within 24 hours. If the cancer patient was depressed and refusing treatment, the nurse navigator would coordinate an appointment with the cancer psychologist. If the cancer patient was in severe pain, the nurse navigator would coordinate a visit with palliative and support care. If the patient had eating problems, the nurse navigator would coordinate the appointment with a dietician and if the patient had problems with transportation to their appointments or paying their hospital bill, the nurse navigator would coordinate a visit with a social worker. Prior to the clinical pathway, the nurse navigators' task completion rate was not tracked. In addition, many tasks were not assigned because the challenge of entering each task for myriad patients became overwhelming. The results were that many cancer patients did not receive the much-needed healthcare required for their survival.

On April 4, 2016, I was doing consulting work at a small hospital, and I saw an elderly Black woman sitting with her head leaning down towards the floor. She looked as though she was in distress. I rushed over to her and asked, "Are you okay. How can I help you?" She raised her head and I immediately recognized her as a member of my church family. For privacy, I will call her, Sister Betty. Sister Betty taught adult Sunday school and was my mother's-in-law good friend for many years. She reluctantly shared that she was recently diagnosed with breast cancer and chose not to tell her family. I was befuddled. She explained that she did not want to be a bother to her only son who lived in Texas or her immediate local family. She had her faith and believed that with God she would fight the monster known as cancer. Surprisingly, this is not uncommon.

Over the years, I have heard stories of myriad cancer patients who do not tell their families of their diagnosis. Sister Betty expressed that she was also exasperated because was going to miss the surgery for her port placement because she did not have transportation. The port was needed for the chemotherapy that she would begin in a week. I asked her if she had a nurse navigator who is responsible for coordinating her appointments, social work, dietary needs, and psychotherapy. She said yes and gave me the name. I knew the nurse navigator and called her immediately. The nurse navigator explained that the surgery was scheduled for 6:00 am the next day and that the patient did not request transportation. I asked Sister Betty if she requested transportation and she said yes. I explained to her and Sister Betty that there must have been a miscommunication. The response of the nurse navigator was very unsettling; she abruptly decided that the resolution was to reschedule the emergency port placement surgery.

At the time, I had several ongoing projects at an ambulatory surgery center including a project to improve surgical case scheduling. I knew that rescheduling Sister Betty's port placement surgery would result in delayed care. That is critical for breast cancer patients to receive timely care. I told the nurse navigator that I would take Sister Betty to her 6:00 am. I remember waking up at 4:00 am to pick up Sister Betty and taking her to the surgery center for her surgery, and then taking her home, after we went to the grocery store to pick up a few things. I could only imagine what would have happened to Sister Betty if God did not put me in the right place at the right time. So, what went wrong? I followed up with the nurse navigator, and she checked the software tool that is used to manage all tasks. Guess what? She admitted that she failed to schedule the transportation for Sister Betty. She apologized and assured me that Sister Betty was in good hands.

Clinical Pathways

A clinical pathway is a tool is employed by healthcare professionals to deliver evidence-based healthcare. Ideally, it ensures that all patients receive healthcare equitably. The supportive care clinical pathway for head, neck, and colorectal cancer patients addresses the software platform challenges with the creation of a nurse navigator checklist. This checklist enables the nurse navigator to quickly select what the patient needs from transportation, dietary, chemotherapy, radiation, and follow-up appointments. In addition, I created a monthly report that not only provided nurse navigator task compliance but also tracked patient demographics and clinical outcomes. The demographics ensured fair access to the new clinical pathway. The results were worthy of the Pathway of the Year Award. The pathway results were outstanding with a decrease in the emergency room rate from 53.6 % to 32.2%, the hospital admission rate from 33.9% to 25.8%, and the 30-day readmission rate from 32.8 % to 20%. As the project leader, I wanted to ensure that Black cancer patients participated in the newly developed clinical pathways.

My role as an internal healthcare consultant allowed me to become a champion for healthcare inequity and access. I had the opportunity to work with many services including emergency, acute care, surgery, cancer, pediatrics, cardiology, infusion centers, palliative care, same-day surgery centers, urgent care, primary care, finance, chronic health, health equity, and patient access. In all of my projects, my goal was to establish care standardizations. Many healthcare protocols are evidence-based, simply meaning that they have been proven and adopted by many institutions. However, many healthcare systems are so complex, that many evidence-based practices are not implemented by all healthcare providers.

As a standardized care delivery consultant, I created training tools for both healthcare providers and patients. It was important to understand the clinical pathway and assign patients who met the eligibility criteria. In addition, I created a reporting system that would measure the following pathway metrics: participation rate by provider and clinical outcomes compared to the goals that would monitor which providers assigned clinical pathways to ensure that all eligible patients had equal access. I remember, shortly after the launch of a new Oncology Patient Clinical Pathway, the participation rate was only 50%. Upon investigation, it was apparent that many oncologists were not assigning the clinical pathway to eligible patients. How were so many patients not meeting the eligibility criteria?

The unfortunate reality is that doctors and nurses are the arbiters of which patients receive indispensable healthcare. Some of the oncologists admitted that they were biased against those cancer patients who did not have transportation. The rationale was that those patients would not be compliant with their scheduled appointments. As a team, we explained to the oncologists that it was crucial for those patients to be assigned the pathway because the nurse navigators would then be able to identify all of the patient's needs including transportation. As the project manager, I reviewed the new pathway training process. I found that there was a training gap. Some providers did not understand the pathway eligibility criteria. Thus, they did not assign the pathway properly. I updated the training materials to clearly define the eligibility criteria. I also added a step for the oncology nurses to check all eligible patients to ensure that the pathway was assigned. After retraining the providers, the pathway participation rate increased to 95%. Thus, helping to keep high-risk cancer patients out of the emergency room and hospital.

As a consultant working on cancer projects, I worked with healthcare providers who were not always aware of their explicit racial bias. Each year, I worked with the Cancer Executive Leadership team on their business strategy and the new initiative based on their annual operating plan deliverables. I was facilitating the annual Strategy Planning meeting with approximately twenty leaders. The leadership team had already agreed on several potential strategic projects. The next strategic deliverable was aligned with health inequity. The team had to choose between the English Second Language Interpreters project or the project for Reducing Black Women's High Risk of Triple Negative Breast Cancer.

One of the white female managers stated emphatically, "We all know why Black women have higher rates of breast cancer. It's because they are all obese." We are in a large conference room, and everyone is seated around a large rectangular table. As the only Black woman in the room, I leaned forward so that she could see me. I asked her to repeat what she had just stated. She turned red and apologized. She agreed that the Triple Negative

Breast Cancer Project was very important and that there was no need to expand the Interpreter program.

While I was gathering my belongings at the end of the meeting, I felt a surge of disappointment at witnessing firsthand blatant discrimination against the resources for a program targeting Black women with the most aggressive form of breast cancer. Triple Negative Breast cancer is very aggressive and Black women have the highest mortality rate at 59% compared to white women at the cancer center. The Cancer Community Outreach manager walked over to me and stated that she wanted to apologize to me personally and that she was not racist. I told her that I was very concerned that she was responsible for community outreach with her explicit bias against Black women with cancer.

As the consultant for the newly formed "Reduce Triple Negative Breast Cancer Project" team, I was responsible for creating the project goals and deliverables. The same Cancer Community Outreach manager who did not want this important project was also on the team. As the team brainstormed the root causes for why Black women did not get genetic counseling, one reason was that there were no Black Community Outreach Coordinators. The manager explained that she never needed Black coordinators because she worked with volunteers from Black sororities.

So, I asked her, "How many coordinators do you have?"

She replied, "I have six total, three Whites, two Hispanics, and one Asian."

I then asked, "Approximately 21% of the cancer center patients are Black, 65% are White, 8% are Hispanic and less than 1% are Asian, do you think that it would be important to have Black coordinators?"

She sighed and stated, "If you have a problem, you should talk to my manager."

I took her advice and within two months, the very first Black community outreach coordinator was hired. The impact was immediate, as more Black women with Triple Negative Breast Cancer were able to talk to an employee versus a volunteer about important health issues. I wonder what would have happened if I was not the only Black healthcare consultant working at the cancer center. Who would look out for the important healthcare needs of Black cancer patients? The fact is that systemic racism is not only cultural but also structural. In the United States, the foundation of cancer research, policies, and programs consistently are developed, implemented, and ran by the majority of white staff. Working as a healthcare consultant for over a decade, in the majority of my meetings with executives, physicians, nurses, and support staff, 99% of the time, I was the only Black leader in the room. It was my responsibility to remind white leaders that health equity for Black patients who are their customers, begins with the acknowledgment of the institutional racism in healthcare delivery.

The Structure of the Healthcare System – It is Complex

Why is the United States of America healthcare so complex? When I first started my journey into the U.S. Healthcare system in the pharmaceutical industry and then healthcare delivery, I learned quickly that it was very complex. I found it quite disconcerting that the dearth of Black leadership in healthcare delivery yielded countrywide health disparities. I wanted to understand the process and created what I named, "The Vicious Cycle of Healthcare Delivery" as shown in figure 2.

In "The Vicious Cycle of Healthcare Delivery" the process starts with the person or the ill patient who is in need of care. For most of us, we would take a quick trip to the drugstore or grocery store for an over- the-counter (OTC) remedy. For some, an at-home remedy is sufficient to address the illness. However, for a more serious illness, a trip to the emergency room, urgent care facility, or doctor's office may be warranted. In those instances, the next step is for the healthcare provider to perform an assessment to gather data about the problem. Is it shortness of breath? Is it abdominal pain? Is it a broken bone? As the patient, this is when you share the problem with the healthcare provider. After the assessment, lab work, imaging, or a consult with a specialist may be ordered. At this point, the goal is to define what the ailment is in the form of the diagnosis. This is the time to have a serious conversation with the provider to understand your options. Also, a time to determine if a second opinion is warranted. After the diagnosis, a treatment plan is created to address the disease. The complexity of healthcare delivery demonstrates how the process can break down at any step. There are also opportunities to exit the vicious cycle with specific "end" steps.

The first endpoint is when the sick person or the "patient" seeks healthcare in the form of an over-the-counter (OTC) or home remedy and recovers fully. The second endpoint occurs when the patient goes to the emergency room (ER) and is sent home without proper treatment. This is very dangerous and can end with death. The third endpoint occurs after the patient's illness or disease has been properly diagnosed and treated with a good patient health outcome. The fourth endpoint is when the vicious cycle continues with poor care healthcare delivery and the patient dies. Thereby, seeking assistance from poor external sources can create more problems and the results can be deadly. I will share my healthcare nightmare shortly.

A hypothetical case is the breast cancer patient, Pauline. She is a Black 37-year-old married mom of three children and works as a teaching assistant. For the past two years, she has seen the same white 55-year-old male doctor who is pleasant yet unengaged. During a recent breast self-exam, Pauline feels a small lump. During her annual check-up, a few weeks later, she mentions the lump to her doctor. He is not actively listening to her findings and does not order a mammogram. Why? For years, the guidelines indicate that women should be eligible for screening mammograms starting at age 40. However, the guideline data is based on white women and does not consider that Black women have the highest breast cancer mortality rate. Unfortunately, Pauline is not screened early for breast cancer. The lump that she felt continues to grow, and a year later, she goes to another physician and is diagnosed with Stage 3 triple negative breast cancer.

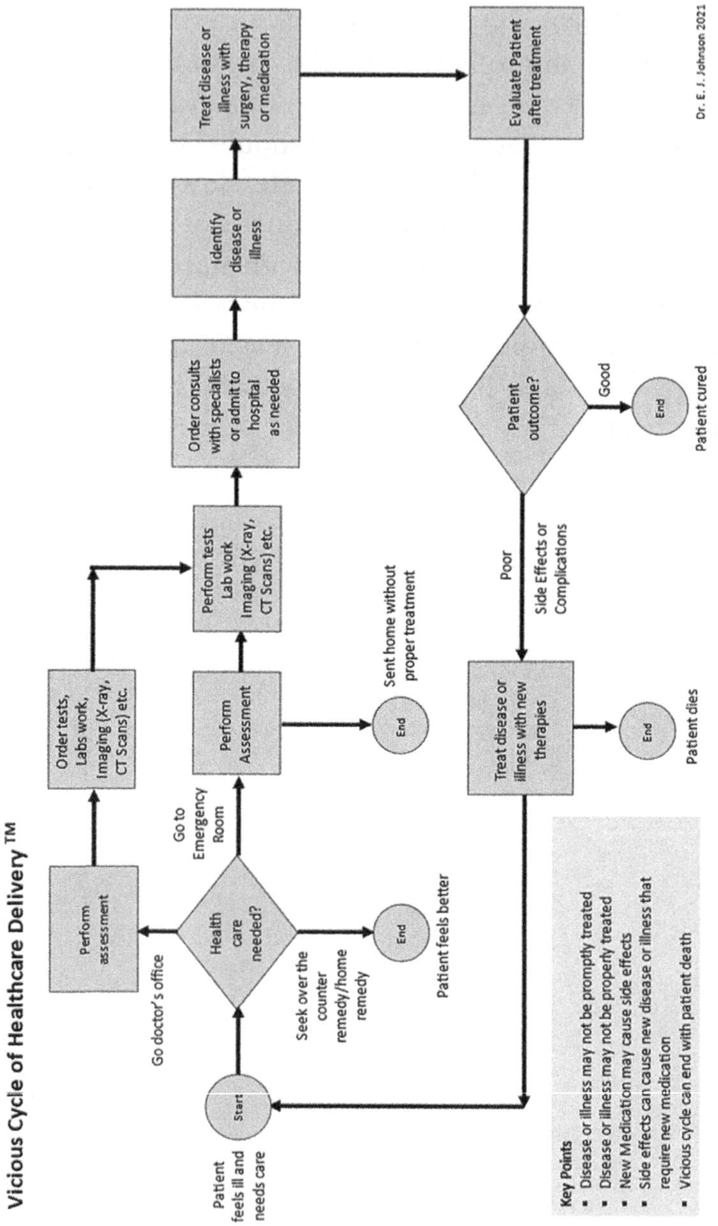

Figure 2 The Vicious Cycle of Healthcare Delivery

Another hypothetical case involves Calvin who has high blood pressure. Calvin is an active Black retired single 69-year-old mechanic with a passion for tennis. He is on Medicare and has seen the same older white physician annually for four years. He was diagnosed with high blood pressure two years ago. However, he was never informed of the life-threatening consequences of high blood pressure including stroke, heart attack, and kidney damage. He was prescribed Lisinopril but does not take it consistently. Nor, does the physician recommend that he monitor his blood pressure at home with a blood pressure cuff (that he could purchase on Amazon for $25) and begin a low salt, low-fat diet. Calvin lives on fast food, after all, he is single and hates to cook. As a result, Calvin's high blood pressure causes a devasting stroke that leaves him paralyzed on the right side of his body. With no local family to help, Calvin now lives in a nursing home.

In both cases, the patients suffer because of poor healthcare. So, what may be the reason? Research studies have proven that a patient that has a trusting relationship with their doctors enable better communication and better outcomes. The vicious cycle of healthcare can have deleterious consequences and so can healthcare payment models.

How Healthcare Payment Impacts Patient Care

Another complexity of healthcare is how payment and billing can impact healthcare delivery. There are three types of payments for healthcare including Government programs (Medicare and Medicaid), private insurance plans (primarily employer-based), and personal payment (out of pocket).

As a healthcare consultant, I found that billing methods are perhaps the most complex. The two billing models employed in America are the traditional fee-for-service (FFS) and the more recent value-based care (VBC) as noted in Table 1 below:

Table 1 Billing Models – Fee-for-Service vs. Value-Based Care

Fee-for-Service (FFS)	Value-Based Care (VBC)	Comments
Cost is based on preset prices	Lower payment costs.	Improving healthcare delivery requires lower costs.
Billing is based on the cost of service	Cost is based on historic prices and the value to the patient.	Controlling the price of healthcare can be achieved with more efficient care models.
Provider is paid for each service	Payment is based on quality, not quantity.	Improving healthcare quality should be the goal not the number of paid services.
Results can include price inflation and redundancy of care (overpayment)	Providers are incentivized to work to better healthcare outcomes.	Better care is provided to the patient with clear healthcare outcomes tied to payment.
Lower patient satisfaction is common	Preferred by Medicaid and Medicare to improve patient satisfaction.	The current trend is to measure patient satisfaction and link that to provider reimbursement. Providers with low patient satisfaction will receive a financial penalty.

The challenges with the fee-for-service model are billing errors and redundancies. An ill patient can be seen by a primary care doctor and specialist. The same bloodwork can be ordered by all the providers which is not only expensive but frustrating for the patient who has to have blood drawn multiple times for the same test. The other example is when the providers knowingly order unnecessary tests that enrich other providers. In the past decade, many healthcare organizations have been selecting value-based Care models. The Affordable Care Act (ACA) was launched in 2010 and was the first major health legislation in over fifty years. The new law required that patients receive value for the care that they received. The Medicare and Medicaid programs began to demand payment that was based on the quality of the care versus the quantity of care. This is an opportunity to improve efficiency and reduce the overcharging for care that can occur with Fee for Service payment models.

Chapter 2 - Key Points to Remember

1. The theoretical definition of healthcare value is a function of quality and service divided by cost.

2. The theoretical healthcare quality equation is a function of provider knowledge, patient knowledge, and patient advocate knowledge divided by the racial bias factor.

3. Neely Fuller, Jr., the founder of the racism/counter racism concept, outlined that white supremacy controls nine areas of people's activity including economics, education, entertainment, labor, law, politics, religion, sex, and war.

4. Dr. Frances Cress Welsing, a noted psychiatrist, recognized the importance of adding "Health" as the tenth people activity that is controlled by white supremacy racism.

5. In the United States, healthcare delivery is predominately controlled by white people from the hospital CEOs to government policymakers resulting in biased and discriminatory practices. The healthcare data shows poorer health outcomes for the Black community.

6. In 1900, 1940, and 2020, the percentage of all Black physicians in the United States, was 1.3%, 2.8%, and 5.8 % respectively which shows slow progress in the past 120 years.

7. The "Vicious Cycle of Healthcare Delivery" demonstrates how the complex healthcare system can compromise the health and quality of life of Black patients.

8. Healthcare delivery is not equitable and Black patients have worse health outcomes compared to their white counterparts.

9. The American healthcare system has evolved from a Fee for Service with payment for each healthcare service to a value-based system that requires providers to receive payments based on the quality of healthcare.

CHAPTER 3: LONG HISTORY OF RACISM IN HEALTHCARE

Understanding Black Citizenship Status in the United States of America from 1619 to 2021

During my undergraduate years at the University of Pittsburgh with my chemical engineering major, I decided to select Black Studies as my minor. I was elated to take every Black Studies course that would fit into my busy 16-credit-per-semester schedule. Although I grew up in a household that had a strong foundation of Black history, including witnessing my parents' campaign for Dick Gregory when he ran for president in 1968, however, I was thirsty for more knowledge. I remember my very first class, Black People in Colonial America. The course was taught by a seasoned professor who was also a practicing Buddhist. He would actually invite the class to his Buddhist temple and wanted to expose us, a group of freshmen (mainly teenagers), to new religious experiences. In the course, the central theme was that for the majority of time since the arrival to the United States, we were not citizens and did not have the same rights that white Americans inherited at birth. In fact, there were laws, codes, and court rulings that legally upheld "enslavement," followed by second-class citizenship. I would argue that America will not be a true democracy until Black people achieve full citizenship in the ten areas of people activities: economics, education, entertainment, labor, law, politics, religion, sex, war, and health.

The Black experience in the United States is correlated to the citizenship status. The first Black people arrived in Jamestown, Virginia in 1619, not as citizens but as indentured servants.[18] This fact is important because it is often reported that the Angolans were "slaves" which is incorrect. The twenty Angolans as stated on the German ship's manifest, were the same as the white indentured servants. The agreement was for indentured servants to provide labor for six to eight years. This however did change in 1640 when a dispute regarding Black indentured servants went to court. In 1640, Virginia courts sentenced a black runaway servant, John Punch, to "serve his said master for the time of his natural Life."[19] That court ruling impacted the status of Black people and changed it from indentured servants to permanently "enslaved". The other colonies followed suit.

What is Enslavement?

The definition of a slave is "a person who is owned by another person and is forced to work for and obey them." [20] The definition of enslave or an enslaved person is making someone into a slave. To most, both words may evoke a similar connotation. However, there is a tremendous difference. [21] The fact is that Africans were captured, kidnapped, placed on ships, transported to colonies (later to be named the United States), and called slaves. In actuality, the act of enslavement is not so simple. It is a very specific process that literally tortures the mind, body, and spirit. A process to dehumanize and break the spirit to fight their enslavement.

A review of Black Citizenship status from 1619 to 2020 demonstrates that although Black people have lived in what is now called the United States of America, we have not had full citizenship rights for very long. [22]

Per Table 2, The Black Citizenship Status from 1619 to 2020, Black Americans have only been recognized with full rights and protections for only 13.65% or 55 years of the 401-year total time period. For 246 years from 1619 to 1865, Black people did not have any citizenship rights except for the 12-year period called "Reconstruction." The Reconstruction era was from 1863 to 1877 which followed the American Civil War. It was during Reconstruction that the 13th, 14th, and 15th amendments were signed into law.

The Thirteenth Amendment to the United States Constitution abolished slavery and involuntary servitude, except as a punishment for a crime. The amendment was passed by Congress on January 31, 1865, and ratified by the required 27 of the then 36 states on December 6, 1865, and proclaimed on December 18, 1865. The Fourteenth Amendment to the United States Constitution, ratified in 1868, granted citizenship to all persons born or naturalized in the United States—including formerly enslaved people—and guaranteed all citizens "equal protection of the laws." However, in the late 1870s, the Southern Republican Party vanished with the end of Reconstruction. The southern states' governments effectively nullified both the 14th Amendment. The Fifteenth Amendment was ratified in 1870 and granted Black men the right to vote. It states that, "The right of citizens of the United States to vote shall not be denied or abridged by the United States or by any State on account of race, color, or previous condition of servitude."[23]

Table 2.

Black Citizenship Status From 1619 to 2021

Time Period	Citizenship Status in years	Percent (%) of U.S. Experien ce	Black Citizenship Status	Key Legal Activities
1619-1865 "Chattel Slavery"	246	61.36%	No citizenship rights or voting rights	• Slaves are legally Property • Black enslaved people are counted as three-fifths human as per the constitution • Citizenship is for whites only • "Slave Codes" are enacted in all colonies • Dred Scott decision declares that enslaved people are not citizens • Trans- Atlantic Slave Trade and Slave breeding begins in the colonies • 1787 US Constitution is ratified by white men of which 80% own "slaves" • White immigration increased to maintain a white majority

1865–1877 Recon-struction Era **Black men get the right to vote**	12	2.99%	Citizenship and voting rights are granted	• "Slavery" is abolished with 13th, 14th, and 15th Amendments signed into law • Freedman's Bureau is established and begins providing funding, education and healthcare to newly freed "slaves;" grant of 40 acres and a mule is launched • Blacks have the right to vote and win elections for Governor, Lt. Governor, Senate, House of Representative, Mayor • President Andrew Jackson supported the nullification
1878–1953 Jim Crow Era **Legal Segregation**	100	24.94%	Limited citizenship rights	• Lynching and Ku Klux Klan terrorism • Legal segregation implemented 1896 • Apartheid, discrimination, institutional racism in effect in all areas of life activities • Redlining prevents Black home ownership • Laws prevent Black business ownership
1953-2008 Civil Rights Era **Fight for Human Dignity**	43	10.72%	Most citizenship rights	• Civil Rights Act (1964) passed • Voting Rights (1965) passed • School desegregation law (1954) is not enforced

New Jim Crow				• No government support for new laws
2009-2020 Fight for Racial Justice Black Lives Matter & Anti-Racism Movements	12	2.93%	Reduction in citizenship rights	• Holder vs Shelby (2013) Voting Rights Bills Pre-Clearance removed • Blatant Voter Suppression laws implemented across the United States • Protests against the murder of George Floyd by police filmed on video has not resulted in new laws
1619-2021	402	100.00%	The struggle for full citizenship continues	

Data compiled from: Brinkley A. The Unfinished-Nation: A Concise History of the American People, New York: Knopf; 1991; Higginbotham A. In the Matter of Color: Race and the American Legal Process: The Colonial Period, New York, Oxford University Press; 1978; Kluger R. Simple justice: The History of Brown v Board of Education and Black America's Struggle for Equality. New York: Knopf; 1976; Marable M. Race, Reform and Rebellion: The Second Reconstruction in Black America, 1945-1990, revised second edition, Jackson: University Press of Mississippi; 1991; Marshall TH. Citizenship, Social Class and Other Essays, Cambridge, England: Cambridge University Press; 1950. https://www.ncbi.nlm.nih.gov/pmc/articles/PMC2593958/

Ironically, the lack of basic citizenship rights was not the precursor to poor healthcare of Black people in the United States. The foundation of the poor healthcare delivery and subsequently poor health outcomes is due to racism.

Healthcare History in the United States by Era

Healthcare During Enslavement

The health of Black people in the United States today can be directly correlated to the health status of enslaved Black people. As a child, my mom would often quip. "That's because we are from strong stock." She shared that Black people throughout the world had to deal with white supremacy racism, and to survive, we had to be strong mentally, physically, and spiritually. I can only imagine the mental trauma of being whipped, raped, beaten, and enduring the painful separation from loved ones. Mental health is, even today, a struggle for many Black people who must deal with intergenerational trauma. Yet her inspiring words remind me of the book that I read decades ago entitled, *Remembering Slavery.* [24] What was amazing was that the book actually had a set of tapes that captured the actual voices of formerly enslaved Black people who were able to tell their personal experiences. These are the only known recordings from the Federal Writers' Project in the 1930s. It is reported that these invaluable tapes were stored in the Library of Congress and prior to the book, simply collecting dust.

The narratives of the enslaved who spoke of the harsh conditions in which they live were gut-wrenching. The story of Papa Dallas is perhaps the most haunting. In their own voice via an actual recording, that was actually included with the book, *Remembering Slavery,* narrates how Black people remembered their lives while enslaved. The story, which is desperately sad, recounted how Papa Dallas, as boy in the early 1800s, had learned how to read. He told the story of how he was caught reading to other enslaved Black people. The wicked plantation owner, called "Massa," upheld the law that made it illegal for Black people to read. Think about this as we try to understand how we had to be from unbelievably "strong stock." It was literally illegal for you to learn how to do something that we take for granted today, the ability to simply read.

The legal response to such an action, for a child who dared to learn how to read, was to be whipped 20 lashes. However, this "Massa" retrieved a poker, placed it in the flames of a wood-burning stove, and Papa Dallas shared in his raspy recorded voice, "he burned my eyes out." The picture of Papa Dallas in the book is seared in my mind forever along with his tragic experience. What healthcare did Papa Dallas receive? Was he immediately rushed the white doctor for the treatment of his horrific injuries that resulted in permanent blindness and terror? No. The healthcare that was rendered during enslavement was essentially provided by the enslaved. Papa Dallas shared his narrative and stated that his mother tended to his care after the assault by the white plantation owner.

The British Empire had thirteen colonies that exploited the free labors of enslaved Black people who worked on cotton, sugar, and tobacco plantations. The kidnapping and transportation of Black people, during the Transatlantic Slave Trade, increased exponentially during the eighteenth century. This was a legal practice in all thirteen colonies.

The health issues of enslaved Africans were widespread due to poor hygiene and diet. It is a myth that enslavers took good care of those that they enslaved for economic reasons. The fact that plantation owners owned humans is a demonstration that they did not have empathy or care for their health needs. The 2014 term "Black Lives Matter" is rooted by the fact that for over four centuries, Black life in America is constantly "devalued, disrespected and marginalized." This is a fact that is shared often by radio talk show host, Joe Madison.

Doctors Were Rare

According to multiple accounts, in the colonies (and future states) the diseases among the enslaved Africans included: typhus, measles, mumps, chicken pox, typhoid, and more. One account stated the following:

> "Only as a last resort did the slave owner bring in a doctor. Instead, the white master and his wife would provide the health care, though rarely were either one [a] trained physician. As with everything else, Blacks had no say about their care. And if a doctor was involved, Black patients were not necessarily told anything about their condition. The medical report went directly to the slave owner." [25]

However, what was more common was for the elder enslaved women to provide healthcare via their knowledge of herbs, roots, and plants. In addition, they brought their midwifery knowledge from West Africa to the colonies. Thereby the role of enslaved Black women was multifaceted. Not only did they toil in the fields, but they also took care of the sick along with their families.

An unfortunate historic milestone occurred in 1808 when the Transatlantic Slave Trade was banned in the United States. Since kidnapped Africans could no longer be purchased and enslaved, the white government structures sanctioned the mass breeding of enslaved Africans. A pregnant enslaved woman contributed to the new labor pool. Regrettably, this new protocol was echoed across the colonies that the birth of a baby born into enslavement meant profits and wealth that potentially lasted for generations.[26] The enslaved woman was now considered a commodity that required little investment including the cost of adequate healthcare. However, the desire to increase the slave population through breeding posed horrific health challenges including infant mortality and many mothers dying during childbirth.

Experimentation on Enslaved Black Women and Infants

The health of the enslaved was always in jeopardy. It is well documented that enslaved Black men and women were used in medical experiments. In the case of the so-called "father of modern gynecology," J. Marion Sims, he was well known for conducting experiments on enslaved Black women without anesthesia or consent, based on a heinous belief that Black people do not feel pain. [27] In this case Sims inflicted tremendous pain on the women, pregnant women, and even infants who sometimes died. Despite the torture of these enslaved women and babies, both the white physicians and white medical institutions gained considerable fame and wealth for decades.

To this day, many white researchers have defended the actions of Sims by stating that enslaved Black women did have "the right" to give consent to have experiments done on them without anesthesia. These absurdly deviant sentiments were echoed in 2021 when a large statue of J. Marion Sims was removed from New York Central Park. However, the true Sims story is even more frightening and disturbing. The question that Dr. Joy DeGruy posited in her book, *Post Traumatic Slave Syndrome*, "So where did Sims get all those women to run his experiments?" is critical in understanding the torture and oppression of the enslaved Black women.

History revealed that Sims actually purchased enslaved Black women from "slave owners" who deemed them as supposedly, "not fit for duty." [28] These women were suffering from an obstetric fistula. This illness is one of the most serious and tragic childbirth injuries to mothers. It is described as a hole between the birth canal and bladder and/or rectum which developed after prolonged, obstructed labor without access to timely, high-quality medical treatment. Thereby, enslaved Black mothers were at a higher risk for this obstetric fistula due to inadequate healthcare. This disorder results in the leakage of urine and / or feces into the vagina which had to be miserable and painful resulting in serious infections. However, this did not interrupt the daily work on the plantation. What work did it preclude? The answer is difficult and sad to contemplate, however it was the "rape" of enslaved Black women who had a body odor due to their ailment. Sims was then able to purchase these "not fit for duty" enslaved women for gynecological experiments. One woman reportedly endured thirty gynecological surgeries without anesthesia by the evil Sims. Thus, adverse health consequences for enslaved Black women facilitated the establishment of some medical advances that are used today, including the invention of the speculum that is used during gynecological exams.

Healthcare During Reconstruction

On March 3, 1865, Congress enacted legislation to establish a Bureau for the Relief of Freedmen and Refugees, commonly known as the Freedmen's Bureau.[29] This agency was founded at the request of President Abraham Lincoln as a way to integrate the recently freed slaves into the fabric of American society. It was felt that affirmative assistance was required to educate, feed, settle, and economically empower the recently freed Black slaves and poor whites after the Civil War. In addition, the bureau was charged with providing emergency and temporary healthcare until state and local authorities could assume this responsibility because of the significantly poor health of these newly freed citizens. High rates of infectious diseases, such as tuberculosis and smallpox, high infant mortality, severe malnutrition, and unaddressed injury were well documented. Despite its efforts during its seven-year existence, the bureau never fully fulfilled its mission because of continued underfunding, political resistance, and overt racism that was the hallmark of Southern resentment during the Reconstruction period.

Black women continued to play a significant role in administering care in these early days of freedom, most notably when it came to childbirth. Mortality in those early days was extremely high, most especially for infants and small children. Malaria was particularly brutal, as was diphtheria and yellow fever. Most of the sick were treated with folk remedies even after the invention of vaccines including smallpox. The dire reality was that there was virtually no government regulation or attention paid to public health that reduced rampant infection of disease.

Healthcare During Jim Crow Apartheid

The Jim Crow Era, less commonly known as "apartheid," was a legal response to the freedom of Black people in the United States from the start of 1877 to the Civil Right Act of 1965. The litany of Black Codes and Jim Crow segregation ensured that the 13th, 14th, and 15th amendments that were established during the Reconstruction Era were nullified. The goal was to effectively maintain de-facto slavery. During this time, the health problems that were present during enslavement continued for the next 100 years. Including healthcare of Black children who would begin plantation work in the fields as young as six years old.[30] The "Black Codes" also known as the "Slave Code" not only forced enslaved Africans to work for free but also essentially placed them under surveillance.[31] Every movement was monitored by the local authorities and the local officials including their travel to meetings and even church services. Enslaved

Black people needed passes and white sponsors to move from place to place or to leave town. Collectively, these regulations codified a permanent underclass status for Black Americans today.

Due to the legal separation of the races in both the northern and southern parts of the country. The need for quality healthcare was desperately needed. The timeline for Slave Codes and Laws is listed in Table 3 below.

Table 3. Timeline of "Slave" Laws and Activities in Colonial Virginia

Year	Law /Activity/Virginia Slave Codes	Impact
1612	First tobacco crop in Jamestown, Virginia	The social exclusion of Black people
1619	The first 20 Black people from Angola, Africa arrive in Jamestown, Virginia as indentured servants	The first Black people are treated the same as White indentured servants
1636	The Colonial North American "slave trade" begins with the launch of a ship named, "Desire"	This is the start of the mass kidnap, capture, and enslavement of Africans in the colonies
1640	John Punch, a runaway Black indentured servant, is sentenced to servitude for life and becomes the first documented "slave."	Whites continue to be indentured servants, but Black people are now "slaves" for life
1680	Runaway "slave' law – Harsh punishment for any "slave" who tried to escape	A form of terrorism to prevent "slaves" from obtaining their freedom

1691	Manumission of "slaves" was not allowed in Virginia, they had to leave the colony	Enabled that only Black people in Virginia were enslaved
1705	Virginia Slave Codes Slave Status – Defines slaves as real estate	The dehumanization of Black people is legal and engrained into society
	Acquits "masters" who kill "slaves" during punishment	White people can kill Black people with impunity
	Forbids "slaves and free-colored peoples" from physically assaulting white people	The hierarchy and the protection of whiteness
	"Slaves" do not have the right to bear arms	The inability of Black people to protect themselves with guns, rifles, etc.
	"Slaves" must have written permission to move abroad	Controls the movement of Black people
1723	Virginia declares manumission illegal	It is illegal for enslaved Blacks to gain their Freedom
1775	The slave population in the colonies is nearly 500,000. In Virginia, the ratio of free colonists to "slaves" is nearly 1:1. In South Carolina it is approximately 1:2	There is a concern that the number of "slaves" in Virginia is equal to free white people
1778	Virginia prohibits the importation of slaves	Virginia leaders want to limit the number of Black "slaves" in Virginia

https://www.thirteen.org/57ent/slavery/timeline/1788.html

After the Black Codes had been enacted throughout the South in 1865, Congress passed the Civil Rights Act of 1866 to give Black Americans limited rights. This legislation allowed Black people to rent or own property, enter contracts and bring cases before courts, only against other Black people. Moreover, it allowed individuals who infringed upon their rights to be sued.[32]

Healthcare During the Civil Rights Era

In 1965, the second Civil Rights Act for Black Americans was passed nearly 100 years after the first Civil Rights Act of 1866. By this time there had been multiple studies and legal challenges that demonstrated the deleterious impact of racism on Black mental, physical, emotional, financial, and spiritual health. It appeared that the measure of Black pain and misery was a key performance indicator of the success of well-designed health policies.

The Jim Crow segregation laws that made it illegal for white nurses to treat Black men, were not immediately mitigated with the passage of the Civil Rights Act which prohibited racial discrimination in employment and education. It also outlawed racial segregation in public places such as hospitals, schools, buses, parks, and public swimming pools. The next important legislation was the 1965 Voting Rights Act which protected the rights of Black American voters and resulted in a backlash of gerrymandering and ongoing voter suppression.

The number of people that died over the years for the passage of the Civil Rights Act and the Voting Rights Act is a testament to the fortitude of the Black men and women who were committed to creating a better future for their children. White leaders had asked if perhaps Black people should leave the United States and go to Africa as recommended by many white leaders including President Abraham Lincoln who wanted all Black people to migrate to Liberia. This view was adopted by some Black leaders including Marcus Garvey who led a movement to return home to Africa. However, leaders including Dr. Martin Luther King were determined to stay in the country built with the free labor of enslaved Black men, women, and children. How would the departure pay homage to the ancestors? Was it possible for a people who were enslaved for 246 years followed by 100 years of Jim Crow to get government support for the new Civil Rights legislation? Could the status of Black people change to include better healthcare? The health status of Black people during the Civil Rights Era did show small signs of improvement.

Healthcare During President Obama's Administration

The Affordable Care Act (ACA) also rebranded as Obamacare by the republicans in 2009, was enabled into law in 2010. The primary goal of the new healthcare policy that was launched in 2010 was to expand healthcare to more Americans. At that time approximately 45 million Americans did not have health insurance. America, the wealthiest country in the world, can easily provide health insurance to every citizen, however, this is not the case. It is important to understand why health insurance for all has been elusive.

The history of health insurance in America is an interesting quagmire of events. The first was the election of Franklin D. Roosevelt as the US president in 1932. After the election, he had an opportunity to pursue universal healthcare coverage for all Americans. Several factors influenced his decision against the idea. The American Medical Association had the strongest opposition. Roosevelt considered nationalizing healthcare as part of his plan for Social Security and was known to be politically astute.[33] He quickly realized that the entanglement of universal health coverage and the Social Security Act would lead to failure for both legislative initiatives.

Of course, Roosevelt's decision left unresolved the pressing need of many Americans for some way to deal with healthcare costs. In the grips of the Great Depression, many were hard-pressed to find the money for essentials like food and shelter. Healthcare often fell by the wayside for families working to access the basic necessities of life.[34] During that time unemployment skyrocketed and health insurance was no longer a priority.

In America, the health insurance industry has similar origins to that of fire insurance. Each system is basically a form of socialism in which the people pay insurance premiums to protect themselves as needed. For example, in the rare instance that a home is engulfed in flames and must be either repaired or replaced by their fire insurance. The health insurance business started with individual insurance plans. Private health insurance like Blue Cross and Blue Shield plans were essential to paving the way for private insurers to meet customer needs. During this time period, employers were not involved in the insurance business since the original health insurance offerings were purchased almost exclusively by individuals. Individuals were able to purchase insurance from an open market, which had competitive pricing.

After the depression, the next big event was World War II. As a result of the war, the fragile economy was on the verge of a total collapse. To combat inflation, the 1942 Stabilization Act, also known as the Emergency Price Control Act, was passed by congress.[35] This act was designed to limit employers' freedom to raise wages and thus to compete on the basis of pay for scarce workers. At the time, there was a quest to find a new way to attract employees. The answer was for employers to offer health benefits as incentives instead of wages. This was a transformational idea in the health insurance industry that soon created the "employee's company" as a new health insurance business This became a tax advantage for employees because health benefits could be considered part of compensation but did not count as income and workers did not have to pay income tax or payroll taxes on those benefits. Thus, by 1943, employers had an increased incentive to make health insurance arrangements for their workers, and the modern era of employer-sponsored health insurance began, a pivotal point in the history of American healthcare.[36]

This change in healthcare was created to be a new incentive to attract new employees. Companies began providing health insurance for not only the employees but also their families. So how did this new insurance plan work? A company was able to purchase a large group health insurance plan at a reduced rate. The company would cut the wages of the employees to cover the health insurance cost. As the years progressed and healthcare costs increased during the year, companies began asking their employees to pay for their health insurance. It was offered as a proposal with the employer paying 50% of the insurance premium. In addition, many employees were offered a sliding scale for their health insurance costs. Higher earners, for example, the corporate CEO, would pay more for their health insurance compared to the same health insurance for the janitor at the same company. How much more money would the American worker earn if they were not tethered to their company's health insurance. Some experts estimate that workers would earn between 4.7% and 31.7% more income if their health insurance was purchased independently like home insurance.[37]

Think about this, as an American, you can go to the open market and purchase car insurance, home insurance, and life insurance. However, most Americans obtain health insurance through their employers. This is not only the tradition but the expectation. One of the major concerns of the new Affordable Care Act (ACA) was that people would not be able to keep their employer-based insurance in lieu of federally controlled healthcare.

My burning question for years has been, should Americans be able to purchase health insurance on the open market in the same way that they purchase automobile insurance, home insurance, and life insurance? The ACA did provide health insurance as an open market for Americans who were self-employed or unemployed and needed insurance for themselves and their families. The number of Americans without health insurance was reduced from 45 million Americans to 20 million Americans.[38] Typically, unemployed, young, and healthy Americans do not buy health insurance. The reason is simple. Why purchase something that I would not use? The same is not true for home insurance and automobile insurance. To qualify for a home loan or even a loan refinance, the lending institution requires proof that the home has been insured. In all fifty states, it is illegal to drive a car that is not insured. There are countless examples of how drivers are sued when they are in car accidents and damage other vehicles. This is currently not true for Americans who do not have health insurance.

So, what is the consequence of playing Russian roulette with your health if you do have appropriate insurance? A car accident or grave illness can eliminate entire savings accounts coupled with debt collections. This financial instability for a family could result in dire consequences. The ACA was able to help millions of Americans afford health insurance. A small penalty was imposed on anyone who failed to enroll in the ACA insurance plan. One of the most important elements of the ACA was insurance premiums that are based on a sliding pay scale (based on income) and a new preventative maintenance program. With the ACA, patients can receive free annual physical exams including mammograms and pap smears. The early cancer screening programs along with physical exams to assess the risks for diabetes, heart disease, and kidney disease is life-changing for many Americans.

The access to affordable health insurance was improved with the expansion of the Medicaid health insurance program to more eligible Americans. The updated Medicaid program allowed states to enroll more people with the Federal government paying for the program for the first three years. After three years, the states would pay 10% of the Medicaid insurance. The Obama Administration was particularly dismayed when many white republican governors from states with larger Black populations, refused to expand their Medicaid programs.[39]

The cultural impact of the ACA on hospitals across the country was also significant. The traditional fee-for-service model was no longer the gold standard. It was being replaced with the new value-based care model. At one time, it was thought that this would be impossible to implement, but many hospitals hired healthcare consultants, like me, to help them with the new requirements.

Healthcare During President Trump's Administration

Donald Trump campaigned with the promise to repeal the Affordable Care Act entirely and replace it with something better. However, once in office congress voted to keep the ACA. However, the Trump Administration was able to damage the efficiency and effectiveness of the ACA law. The penalty for not having some form of health insurance was removed and the marketing budget for the October ACA enrollment campaign was severely reduced. The impact was millions of Americans who were eligible for the ACA would not have access. The corporate response was to raise the co-pay and deductible for employees.

In December 2019, the Trump administration was informed about the pending global pandemic, SARS COVID-19. This was a novel virus with the first documented case discovered overseas.[40] The Obama Administration had successfully responded to the Avian flu virus and the Ebola virus. I remember the international response to the Avian Flu virus. It was 2009, and I was in Manchester, England waiting to board a flight to the United States. I was working for a British company and had attended a week of meetings with my global team. There was an announcement stating that due to the global pandemic, Avian flu, all flights in and out would be suspended. I was fortunate in that my flight was the last flight to the United States. I was relieved to arrive home. At the time, Vice President Biden was responsible for leading the global pandemic response. His team created a Global Pandemic Playbook, and actually left a copy of the playbook for the Trump Administration. The playbook was not used. Instead, the Trump Administration did not have an expeditious response to the COVID -19 virus. Instead, the American people were told that the virus was not serious and that it would go away quickly. Unfortunately, in the three months in which the global pandemic playbook was not reviewed by the Trump [administration], the healthcare of hundreds of millions of Americans would be in jeopardy.[41] This new global pandemic soon came closer to my home.

On March 8, 2020, my husband came home from work early. As a healthcare consultant, I was working from home and was surprised when I heard the door open. He informed me that one of his co-workers tested positive for the SARS-2 coronavirus and that he was told to quarantine for 14 days. I checked the state's COVID-19 website, and his colleague was the 8th person in our state to test positive. This was now very serious and my husband and I were at risk. At the time, he did not have any symptoms and self-isolated to our guest bedroom. As a consultant, I was able to see the COVID-19 hospital data from various institutions. It was frightening. Not only did Black people have a high rate of contracting the COVID-19 virus, but the death rate was also higher. My husband was blessed, and he never developed any symptoms. He was required to have two negative COVID-19 tests before he could return to work. I held my breath each and every day that he left for work as an essential city employee during the early days of the global pandemic.

Why was it Necessary to Shutdown Businesses, Schools, Churches, etc. During COVD-19?

The number of hospitals and healthcare workers in the country had been declining for the last two decades.[42] Some hospital systems had merged to stay afloat, while many had closed their doors permanently. A hospital has a fixed number of hospital beds and staff. In addition, a hospital has a fixed number of life-saving ventilators that are needed to help patients who cannot breathe independently. Due to the limited number of hospital beds and equipment needed to treat all Americans infected by COVID-19, the response was to shut down businesses, schools, and churches. However, hospitals remained open along with home health services.

The data scientists had created COVID-19 models that calculated both infection and death rates. Initially, the data was presented without demographics. However, in May 2020, the news reports began showing the racial disparities of the novel virus. I remember watching the comedian Amber Ruffin on the April 15th, 2020 *Late Night with Seth Meyers* show, entitled, "Amber's Minute of Fury." She admonished the Surgeon General, Dr. Jerome Adams for blaming Black and Brown people for the spread of the COVID-19 virus. She was disappointed that he was espousing Republican talking points. However, her most profound point was that now that it was essentially published that Black and Hispanic people were disproportionately impacted by COVID-19, would white people care enough to take action? She added that if people who went to J Crew were contracting the virus at higher rates, would more be done to address the pandemic? In some cases, white news anchors had guests on their programs that inferred that it was patriotic for older Americans to sacrifice their lives and keep the country open. Thus, if only Black and Hispanic people were dying at higher rates, the small numbers of white people dying would be collateral damage.

The medical community provided COVID-19 education to help save lives. The use of virtual Zoom meetings for Black business owners including barber shops, hair salons, community centers, and churches, served to spread the message of social distancing and mask-wearing. Effective communication was critical to saving the lives of Black people who were at risk of contracting the deadly COVID-19 virus.

What Happened to Healthcare for Black People During COVID-19?

As a healthcare consultant, I worked on myriad projects to set up the new COVID-19 healthcare delivery model. As hospitals prepared for the increase of COVID-19 patients, elective surgery, and office visits were suspended. The volume of patients in the ER dropped precipitously due to the fear of being exposed to COVID-19. The healthcare system began approving new delivery systems including telehealth visits. The goal was to keep people safe. As I consulted with teams to conduct telehealth visits, I learned that many Black households did not have internet access. Thereby, the iPad that they were to receive for their telehealth visit was useless. I asked what would be done to address the gap in care delivery. There was no incentive to address the huge care delivery disparity for those Black patients who could not participate in the newly approved technology.

In the fall of 2020, many healthcare systems could no longer afford to keep the doors closed to elective surgery which is a large revenue source. However, the biggest risk to Black health was patients who did get to see their doctor during COVID-19. Due to missed annual visits, many Black patients did not receive their annual screenings for breast cancer, cervical cancer, lung cancer along with annual blood tests for diabetes and kidney disease, heart disease. It was imperative for primary care physician offices to contact their high-risk patients to let them know that they could be seen in the office. In preparation for medical visits during the COVID-19 pandemic, medical offices were redesigned to allow appropriate social distancing. In addition, frequent hand washing and mandatory face masking became the new normal for public safety.

COVID-19 and Emergency Room Visits

Since the global pandemic began, many Black people have sought emergency treatment for their COVID-19 symptoms. However, sometimes we may not understand what constitutes an emergency. There are two perspectives to consider. The first is from the patient. The American College of Emergency Physicians defines emergency services as follows: "Emergency services are those healthcare services provided to evaluate and treat medical conditions of recent onset and severity that would lead a prudent layperson, possessing an average knowledge of medicine and health, to believe that urgent and/or unscheduled medical care is required." [43] So, two components that should be considered, evaluation and treatment. The second perspective is from the healthcare provider. The provider sees the emergency as determined by the Emergency Department Triage team. It is the triage nurse who is responsible for conducting a brief evaluation based on the patient's complaint. If you find yourself in the needed of emergency health services, it will be essential for you to be prepared.

Preparing for your visit to the Emergency Room

When you arrive at the emergency room, your doctor will ask you many questions about your pain and other symptoms. Remember that answering questions may be difficult if you are in pain, so your doctor will likely give you pain medication. Therefore, if possible, it is important to bring someone with you that knows your health history and how your recent condition has progressed. If you cannot bring someone with you, write down your symptoms to help you remember. You should always have a card with you that lists your allergies, other known conditions, and the medicines you take. The first step of your emergency room visit is an assessment by the triage team.

What is Triage?

In the Emergency Room, all patients are assessed by the triage team. In my case, it was a registered nurse. This process is referred to as triage, which is derived from the French verb *trier*, meaning to separate, sort, sift, or select.[44] Triage is the sorting and prioritization process of determining the severity of a patient's condition. Patients with the most severe emergencies receive immediate treatment. That is why some patients may receive medical care before you, even if they arrived at the emergency room after you. In American emergency rooms, the patients are assigned emergency severity index (ESI) levels as shown in Table 4. [45]

Table 4.

Emergency Severity Index (ESI)

ESI Level	Category	Description	Examples
1	Immediate: life-threatening	Immediate, life-saving intervention required without delay	Cardiac arrest Massive bleeding
2	Emergency: could be life-threatening	High risk of deterioration, or signs of a time-critical problem	Cardiac-related chest pain Asthma attack
3	Urgent: not life-threatening	Stable, with multiple types of resources needed to investigate or treat (such as lab tests plus X-ray imaging)	Abdominal pain High fever with cough
4	Semi-urgent: not life-threatening	Stable, with only one type of resource anticipated (such as only an X-ray, or only sutures)	Simple laceration Pain on urination
5	Non-urgent: needs treatment as time permits	Stable, with no resources anticipated except oral or topical medications, or prescriptions	Rash Prescription refill

In the United States, there are over 130 million visits to the emergency room or emergency departments each year as shown in Table 5.[46] The sad reality is that many Black patients have longer wait times in the emergency room and will leave without treatment. The data for this is often erroneous, because today, many patients provide insurance information or pay in advance during their arrival and may leave without treatment due to long wait times.

Table 5.

2018 Data for Emergency Room Visits in the USA, CDC (Center for Disease Control and Prevention)

Description	Quantity	Percentage of Total
Number of visits	130.0 million	
Number of injury-related visits	35.0 million	26.9%
Number of visits per 100 persons	40.4 million	
Number of emergency department visits resulting in hospital admission	16.2 million	12.5%
Number of emergency department visits resulting in admission to critical care unit	2.3 million	1.8%
Visits with patient seen in fewer than 15 minutes		43.5%
Visits resulting in hospital admission		12.4%
Visits resulting in transfer to a different (psychiatric or other) hospital		2.3%

Unlike the United States, Emergency Departments in other countries have a time requirement for the patient to see a doctor for each Emergency Level. [47]

Table 6. Five Level Triage Systems in Other Countries

System	Countries	Emergency Level	Emergency Level Description	Patient should be seen by doctor within
Australian Triage Scale (ATS)	Australia New Zealand	1 2 3 4 5	Resuscitation Emergency Urgent Semi-urgent Non-urgent	0 minutes 10 minutes 30 minutes 60 minutes 120 minutes
Manchester	England Scotland	1 2 3 4 5	Immediate Very Urgent Urgent Standard Non-urgent	0 minutes 10 minutes 60 minutes 120 minutes 240 minutes
Canadian Triage and Acuity Scale (CTAS)	Canada	1 2 3 4 5	Resuscitation Emergent Urgent Less Urgent Non-urgent	0 minutes 15 minutes 30 minutes 60 minutes 120 minutes

Regardless of triage level or category, in a triage system, the emergency department triage team can decide if emergency care is unnecessary. Since the arrival of the COVID-19 global pandemic in December 2019, the Black community continues to be denied urgent care. In the 8/4/2020 blog post by Dr. Vanessa Grubbs, entitled, "The Health Care System Has the Black Community in a Choke Hold." She reviewed the vicious murders of both

Eric Gardiner and George Floyd who both professed, "I can't breathe." She writes:

> "And now we are hearing it from Black people at the mercy of the American health care system. A system that is literally supposed to help those who can't breathe is figuratively applying a choke hold to Black people by sending them home to die when they say, "I can't breathe." Gary Fowler, a 56-year-old Blackman, was denied COVID-19 testing and hospital admission by three Detroit emergency rooms where he complained of difficulty breathing. Deshaun Taylor, a 23-year-old Black man, was sent home twice from a Chicago hospital, even after testing positive. Reginald Relf, a 50-year-old Black man, was turned away from an urgent care clinic in suburban Chicago without being tested in spite of his labored breathing, fever, and cough. Kimora Lynum, a 9-year-old Black girl with a fever of 103 degrees, was sent home from a Florida academic medical center without being tested. They all died soon after."[48]

These are examples of how during triage, Black patients are denied care.

Black Doctors Matter

I found it interesting that after the murder of George Floyd by a white Minneapolis police officer, Derek Chauvin, there was a meaningful conversation about why "Black Lives Matter?" At the hospitals that I consulted, there were active demonstrations to support the national retort. At one hospital, I participated in the demonstration in which a healthcare worker kneeled for 8 minutes and 41 seconds, (actually 9 minutes and 29 seconds) which is the same time that the convicted officer had his knee on George Floyd's neck. What I found most disconcerting was that the same hospital system had not taken aggressive action to address systemic racism including the hiring and retention of Black physicians. As a consultant at that same hospital, I never met a Black physician, Black nurse, or Black leader. The few Black employees that I met, which was rare, were all in roles in which they "pushed things." They pushed brooms, mops, stretchers, carts, and wheelchairs. When I asked the Black staff why there was a dearth of Black leaders, the response was that white leaders did not want to hire Black healthcare providers. Well, so much for the white leader's commitment to the "Black Live Matters" movement for equality and justice.

A biennial study conducted in 2018 by the Association of American Medical Colleges identified important statistics including the fact that only 5% of physicians in the U.S. are Black or African American, compared to 56.2% of U.S. physicians who are white. While the interest in health-related careers among Blacks and African Americans in the U.S. has increased in recent years, with the Association of American Medical Colleges reporting that 10.5% of students entering medical schools across the country in 2020 are Black or African American, only 3.6% of medical school faculty are Black or African American. The challenge is, what if you only have 5% of physicians who are Black American, and you need medical school professors? In 2018, only 1.5% of the medical school's professors were Black men and only 0.26% are Black women.[49] It is the dearth of Black doctors in America that exacerbates the problem of poor healthcare and the intergenerational trauma due to four centuries of systemic racism and discrimination.

Table 7.

2018 Percentage of Active United States Physicians by Race and Ethnicity vs US Population

Physician Race or Ethnicity	# Physicians	% Physicians	# US Population	% of US Population	Delta
White	516,304	56.2%	197,546,407	60%	-4.2%
Hispanic	53,526	5.8%	59,871,746	18%	-12.5%
Black or African American	45,534	5.0%	40,902,223	13%	-7.5%
Asian	157,025	17.1%	18,728,675	6%	11.4%
Two or More Races	8,932	1.0%	7,114,666	2%	-1.2%
American Indian and Alaska Native	2,570	0.3%	2,417,371	1%	-0.5%
Native Hawaiian or Other Pacific Islander	941	0.1%	586,346	0%	-0.1%
Other	7,871	0.9%	-	0%	0.9%
Unknown	126,144	13.7%	-	0%	13.7%
Total	918,847	100.0%	327,167,434	100%	0.0%

https://www.aamc.org/data-reports/workforce/interactive-data/figure-18-percentage-all-active-physicians-race/ethnicity-2018

The Trauma of Enslavement is Intergenerational

The trauma of enslavement for Black people in the United States is intergenerational or what some refer to as historical trauma; multigenerational trauma; or secondary traumatization. The American Psychological Association's definition of intergenerational trauma is as follows:

> "A phenomenon in which the descendants of a person who has experienced a terrifying event show adverse emotional and behavioral reactions to the event that are similar to those of the person himself or herself. These reactions vary by generation but often include shame, increased anxiety and guilt, a heightened sense of vulnerability and helplessness, low self-esteem, depression, suicidality, substance abuse, dissociation, hypervigilance, intrusive thoughts, difficulty with relationships and attachment to others, difficulty in regulating aggression, and extreme reactivity to stress. The exact mechanisms of the phenomenon remain unknown but are believed to involve effects on relationship skills, personal behavior, and attitudes and beliefs that affect subsequent generations. The role of parental communication about the event and the nature of family functioning appears to be particularly important in trauma transmission. Research on intergenerational trauma concentrated initially on the children, grandchildren, and great-grandchildren of survivors of the Holocaust and Japanese American internment camps, but it has now broadened to include American Indian tribes, the families of Vietnam War veterans, and others." [50]

The important "others" included the Black Holocaust named "American Slavery." It is a challenge for me to fully comprehend how any Black person in America can be mentally healthy. The year 2020 was extremely hard for me and the Black community. There was the constant streaming of dead Black bodies that were murdered by the police or in the case of Ahmaud Arbery, by three white racist vigilantes on all digital platforms. The videos that were on a loop became a form of what some have labeled "Black trauma porn." For some of my friends and family, they tried their best not to partake in this new form of horrific "infotainment."

The intergenerational trauma harkens back to the horrific images of the over 4,000 lynchings of Black men and women across the United States. The gross images were often captured by camera and placed on postcards that were mailed around the world. This trauma of terrorism creates the framework of how Black people must navigate life in America. The goal is to somehow survive both mentally and physically in a country that has yet to fully acknowledge your full humanity. The lived experiences of Black people must include the mental health struggles that are often buried so deeply that they have become normal. The code-switching that occurs between literally two worlds; one white and one Black is considered normal.

As a tutor, I was constantly working with Black students who went to predominately white high schools and shared their stories of feeling out of place. I explained the schizophrenic nature of code-switching that requires one to behave as one person at home and a completely different person when at work or school must be mentally draining. I remember the pain that I felt when I witnessed the mental breakdown of a student who desperately sought white validation and acceptance to only be reminded of the invisible "Whites Only" moniker in their inner circles that forbade her entry. Despite the slow progress achieved over the years, racism continues to have an impact on the mental health of Black people. The negative stereotypes and attitudes of rejection continue to occur with adverse consequences. Historical and contemporary instances of negative treatment have led to a mistrust of white authorities, many of whom are not seen as having the best interests of Black Americans in mind. Since the global COVID-19 pandemic, the mental health needs of Black Americans have increased significantly. However, data shows that when Black people seek mental health support, there are not enough Black psychologists and therapists to meet the demand.

Mental Health and Racism – The Stress Can Kill You

I presume that Black Americans are part of the "others" which the APA failed to include specifically despite the myriad research on the intergenerational trauma from 400 years of enslavement and psychological oppression. However, the "Apology to People of Color for APA's Role in Promoting, Perpetuating, and Failing to Challenge Racism, Racial Discrimination, and Human Hierarchy in the U.S." was a resolution that was adopted by the APA Council of Representatives on October 29, 2021. This was a long overdue apology with the following key points: [51]

1. The APA was complicit in contributing to systemic inequities.

2. The APA hurt many through racism, racial discrimination, and the denigration of people of color.

3. The APA fell short of its mission as an organization to benefit society and improve lives.

4. The APA is profoundly sorry and should have apologized before today.

5. The APA has a shared commitment to assess the harms and those harmed and take responsibility.

6. The APA recognizes that many existing historical records and narratives have been centered around whiteness.

7. The APA resolution is based on a narrative from APA listening sessions, surveys, and historical findings.

8. The APA acknowledges that the harm will continue unless there are interventions that ensure reconciliation, repair, and renewal.

In addition to the formal resolution of apology, the APA also shared with the public, a proposal for a second resolution. The second proposed resolution is entitled, "Psychology's Role in Dismantling Systemic Racism." This resolution includes methods of how psychological science can be instrumental in addressing past harms in practice. The domains would include but are not limited to education, criminal justice, and training. The key points of this proposed comprehensive resolution are noted below: [52]

1. The APA acknowledges that the early history of psychology that was created in the mid-19th century was rooted in the "oppressive psychological science to protect whiteness."

2. The APA confirms that U. S. psychology was developed under the condition of "White epistemologies" that were sustained in research publications that conformed with the white racial hierarchy.

3. The APA was created by white male leadership which contributed to research methods that perpetuated systemic racial oppression.

4. The APA leadership promoted the ideas of early 20th-century eugenics. "*Eugenics is defined as the idea that racial differences and hierarchies are biologically based and fixed, and was used to support segregation, sterilization, and anti-marriage laws.*" As a result, the field of psychology adopted eugenicists conceptual measure of intelligence, health, and capability and then used it to systematically create "the ideology of white supremacy." This racial hierarchy is responsible for the institutional systems that have contributed to not only the financial wealth gap but to the social class disparities.

5. The APA will be proactive and denunciate racism moving forward and design and implement antiracist research using a framework that acknowledges and understands the four levels of racism: structural racism, institutional racism, interpersonal racism, and internalized racism.[7]

6. The APA adopted a framework that affirms that not only is racism a violation of human rights but also stipulates those human rights are both universal and inalienable.

7. The APA must oppose all forms of racism and implement an EDI (Equity, Diversity & Inclusion) framework that will promote psychological safety and emotional intelligence throughout the organization.

8. The APA acknowledges that recent acts of racism have prompted a national discussion about long-standing racial inequities and injustices based on racism, bigotry, and xenophobia.

9. The APA purports that the field of psychology has not historically supported research on communities of color. This included minimal data inclusion and the poor interpretation of results that were biased due to Eurocentric research standards. The ultimate results were the

elevation of white researchers who became the experts in the racially diverse study group.

10. The APA acknowledges the harm to the Black community due to the minimizing of the contributions made by Black psychologists that led to the formation of the independent Association of Black Psychologists (ABPs).

The APA's public apology regarding its failure to challenge racism, racial discrimination, and human hierarchy was an important step. It will take decades of work to address the shortage of Black psychologists, and the long history of racial inequities and injustices. The next step of the APA will be to promote their new anti-racism resolution with a bold strategic plan with specific and measurable goals.

Chapter 3 - Key Points to Remember

1. Black citizenship status has changed from 1619 to 2021 during the period of "Chattel Slavery" to the 2020 Anti-Racism and Black Lives Matter Movement with the passage of constitutional amendments and state laws including voter suppression laws.

2. Healthcare during the enslavement did not address catastrophic health issues that resulted from poor hygiene and diet along with physical trauma from brutal beatings, rape, and torture.

3. The so-called father of modern gynecology, J. Marion Sim performed myriad experiments on enslaved Black women and children without anesthesia or consent resulting in medical advances that benefitted white women.

4. During reconstruction, congress enacted legislation to establish the Freedman's Bureau. The bureau was charged with providing healthcare to newly freed slaves and addressed malnutrition, tuberculosis, smallpox, malaria, and yellow fever. However, the Freedman's Bureau which existed for only seven years was not able to fully fulfill its mention due to resentment and overtly racist congressional actions.

5. The "Slave Laws" and "Black codes" that were first enacted in 1612 provided legal cover for murder, and dehumanization, and established the hierarchy to protect whiteness.

6. In 1942 private health insurance was replaced with employer-based health insurance and was seen as an attractive employee benefit.

7. The Obama administration launched the Affordable Care Act (ACA) and health insurance was once again available on an open market. The ACA also provided preventative maintenance health programs including free annual physicals and cancer screening programs.

8. The Trump administration did not support the ACA and worked to repeal it unsuccessfully. In addition, the administration's poor response to the 2019 global COVID-19 pandemic resulted in a high death rate for Black people across the United States due to racial bias in healthcare delivery.

9. The trauma of enslavement for Black people in the United States is intergenerational. The current shortage of Black doctors, specifically psychologists, makes it nearly impossible to address the mental health needs of the Black community.

10. On October 29, 2021, the American Psychological Association issued a public apology and resolution to people of color for their failure to address, racism, racial discrimination, and the human hierarchy. This is hopefully the first step to creating a strategic and measurable action plan to ameliorate racism, racial discrimination, and the human hierarchy in America.

CHAPTER 4: MEASURING RACISM IN HEALTHCARE USING HEALTH EQUITY

Understanding Health Equity

Health Equity is a term that originated in the 1990s in discussions regarding the impact of institutional racism in healthcare delivery systems. It is defined as follows:

> "Health equity is when all members of society enjoy a fair and just opportunity to be as healthy as possible. Public health policies and programs centered around the specific needs of communities can promote health equity." [53]

However, when health equity is not employed, the result is health inequity. The World Health Organization (WHO) defines health inequity as follows:

> "Health inequity is due to human-made systems and structures that privilege certain groups and underserve or actively oppress others. This occurs through the unequal distribution of power and resources." [54]

In America, poverty can be the result of unfair political and economic systems. People that live in impoverished areas may have reduced access to safe housing, clean water, healthy food, education, and medical care; all can impact health. [50] Health inequity is found across the world and can be addressed on both local and national levels. It can be attributed to human-made systems and structures that privilege certain groups and underserve or actively oppress others. This is a result of the unequal distribution of power and resources as listed in Table 8.[54]

For all types of inequities, there can be intersectionality that can worsen the healthcare situation. It is now more thoroughly understood that a poor Black woman will experience more health discrimination, now place the Haitian woman in a wheelchair who speaks French, you can only imagine how her situation is even worse. I was consulting at a cancer center and attended a meeting with leadership. The issue was a woman from Kenya who was diagnosed with breast cancer. The leaders were discussing the need for her to pay for her healthcare prior to treatment. I asked them if this was normal. Once again, the reaction, was "How did they let her in the room?" The team then agreed that the normal protocol for all cancer patients regardless of country of origin was to complete the consultation and discuss treatment options. Then, and only after the consult, should the patient payment be discussed.

Table 8.

Health Inequities by Type[54]

Health Inequity Type	Description
Racism	A system where one race has the power to control the resources by one race over another, typically meaning that historically marginalized racial or ethnic groups — such as Black, Indigenous, Latinx, Asian, and Pacific Islander
Sexism	A system that privileges one gender over another, meaning that in most cases, men have more privileges than women and other gender identities
Classism	A system that gives unfair advantage to those with wealth and social status and disadvantages those with less
Xenophobia	A system that gives nonimmigrants more power and rights than immigrants
Ableism	A system that values able-bodied people and devalues people with mental or physical disabilities

The systems that create health inequities are often interpreted as complex and interdependent with three levels:[54]

1. Institutional level – this includes how organizations and governments set their laws, policies, and practices that impact how people live.

2. Interpersonal level – this includes how people behave toward each other to ensure equity.

3. Internal level – this includes how people view themselves in relation to one another.

The result of this is environmental, social, and economic differences that impact people's health, which is what leads to health inequity.

Racist Foundation of the Social Determinants of Healthcare (SDOH)

Research demonstrates that there is a difference between good health and access to quality healthcare. There are socioeconomic factors that span over an individual's life that account for as much as 80% of their health. The term "social determinants of health" refers to the environments in which people are born, grow, live, work, and die. Think about it. Your health challenges did not begin with your first visit to your doctor's office or being transported to the emergency room by ambulance. Your healthcare actually began in your mother's womb. It continued with your environment, your community, and the economic stability of your family. How you grew up and who you became as an adult, contributes to your health. The foundation of the Social Determinants of Health is institutional or systemic racism (see Figure 3.)

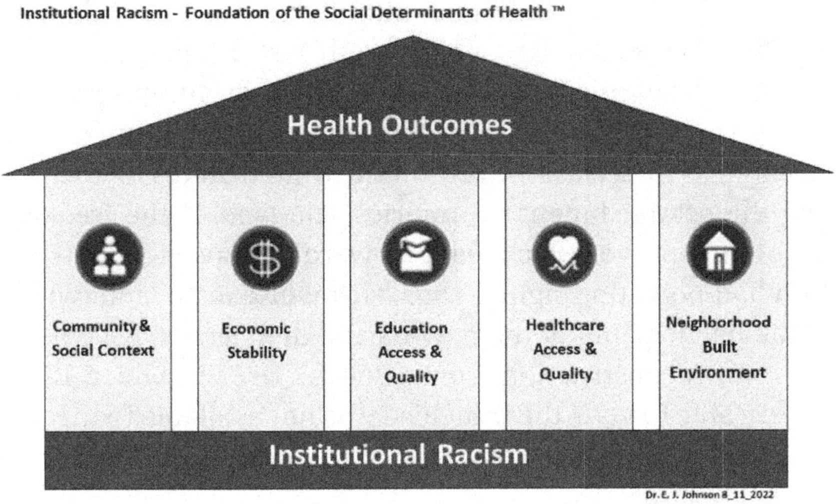

Figure 3 Institutional Racism – Foundation of the Social Determinants of Health

The Social Determinants of Health have institutional racism as its extremely strong foundation. For the last 401 years, in both colonial and ratified United States, Black people have not had full autonomy or control of the socio-economic factors that contribute to their health outcomes. Again, myriad health institutions including the Robert Woods Johnson Institutes estimate that the Social Determinates of Health are responsible for 80% of a person's health outcome. Thereby understanding how racism impacts the most common pillars of the Social Determinants of Health (SDOH) is essential to assessing and solving health disparities. The pillars are outlined below.

1. Community and Social (Political) Context Pillar

The impact of institutional racism on the Black community is profound. The Black community, although not a monolith, with 46.8 million dispersed across the country, still experiences racism similarly regardless of economic status, education, or neighborhood. The Black community, for centuries, fought to be seen and treated as first-class citizens in the United States to no avail. During the establishment of America, the land of the free and home of the brave, Black people were enslaved, and white women had no voting rights. Thus, rich white male landowners were the participants of the new partial democracy. Except the 12 years of reconstruction from 1864 to 1877 in which Black men were able to vote, the franchise was not available to the majority of Black men and women until the passage of the Voting Rights Act of 1965.

Thus, America has only been a true democracy for 57 years. This fact is about to be upended due to the growing white backlash against the "Browning of America." This new adage was adopted recently due to the growing "minority" population and the forecast that in 2050, white people will become a "minority." I wonder how true this will be with the "changing" definition of whiteness. It is plausible that all Hispanics will be categorized as "white" to secure the white majority vote? According to the 2010 census, 53% of Hispanics identified as white in contrast to only 20% in the 2020 census.[55] The fear of the shrinking white American majority is real.

Since the 2020 Presidential election, more than a dozen states have passed countless laws to suppress the votes of the Black community. This is the backlash from the 95% of Black women and 87% of Black men that voted for Joe Biden. To no surprise, in contrast, only 46% of white women and 40% of white men voted for Joe Biden. Yes, contrary to popular opinion, the majority of white women voted for Donald Trump in both 2016 and 2020. The fact is that for the last 50 years, in the past 12 presidential elections, the white vote has been solidly republican with President Obama receiving a mere 43% and 39% of the white vote in 2008 and 2012 respectively. This is juxtaposed to President Obama overwhelmingly receiving 98% of the Black vote in 2008, and 95% of the Black vote in 2012.[56]

Why is this important? The fact is that in the United States, white controlled institutions, whether public or private, have not consistently supported the needs of the Black community since its inception. Therefore, the lack of government funding can be devastating to a struggling community. The research data indicates that in 2021, federal grant funding to Black community nonprofits is paltry at only 1.8% of the total. [57] A good example of the disparate distribution of public funds is how the government and social systems responded to substance abuse.

In the 1980s the Black community was ravaged by the crack cocaine epidemic that continued through the 1990s. Although, drug addiction is a disease, Black victims were met with intense over-policing, and criminalization, followed by mass incarcerations by anyone associated with drugs instead of treatment. I will never forget the *Emerge* cover story of Kemba Smith, a Hampton University student, who in 1994 was sentenced to 24.5 years in prison for being the girlfriend of a major crack cocaine drug dealer, Peter Hall. [58] Although Kemba, never used or handled drugs, she was charged and sentenced as if she was the drug dealer. What I remember as being truly disturbing in the article, entitled, "Kemba's Nightmare," was how incarcerated pregnant Black women are treated. Kemba was pregnant when she entered prison and was handcuffed to her hospital bed after the delivery of her baby boy. This horrendous practice that forces pregnant women to remain in shackles, before, during, and after they give birth is allowed in twenty-three states. This practice is also allowed in the Federal Bureau of Prisons. The crack-cocaine epidemic destroyed Black families for generations.

In contrast, the government and social response to the opioid epidemic which has devastated the white community has been met with government funding and support programs. I remember attending a hospital leadership strategy meeting, and everyone was warned that the new language for opioid addiction was now "substance use disorder" or SUD.[59] The new terminology was to reduce the stigma of drug addiction. The white drug abusers were not arrested, nor were they jailed, and they went to drug rehabilitation centers. It would be wonderful if all communities received the same resources and social support needed for all people to thrive in the places where they live, work, learn, and play. This would have a profound effect on the health of the Black community.

2. Economic Stability Pillar

It is often stated that the United States is the richest country in the world. A decadent display of wealth was highlighted in 2021, with three billionaires, Jeff Bezos, Elon Musk, and Richard Branson launching their respective spaceships into earth's orbit at a cost of billions.[60] When viewing each spectacle, I pondered, how could those billions be used to serve humanity? According to *Fortune Daily*, Jeff Bezos alone has spent at least 5.5 billion dollars for his space venture. [61]

The United States statistics on poverty rate show an increase from 10.5% in 2019 to 11.4% in 2020, which represents 37.2 million people. [62] The annual poverty in the United States could easily be eradicated at an estimated cost of 4.1 billion dollars. Historically, Black Americans have always had the highest poverty rate compared to whites and other racial groups. In 2020, the fact remains with the Black poverty rate at 19.5%, meaning that approximately, 1 out of 5 Black people live in poverty. This is compared to only a white poverty rate of only 8.2% as shown in Figure 4.[62] When people live in poverty, it can be a challenge to afford what most consider, basic necessities such as healthy foods, healthcare, and housing.

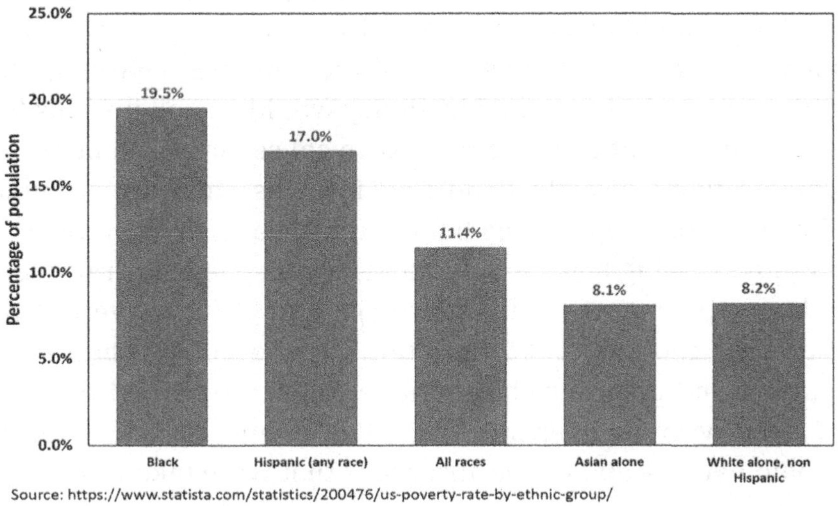

Figure 4 Poverty rate in the United States in 2020 by ethnic group https://www.statista.com/statistics/200476/us-poverty-rate-by-ethnic-group/

In 2021, due to the global pandemic, the democrats without republican support voted and passed the CARES Act which provided temporary relief to struggling families. The act provided families with $300 per month for every child under 6 years old and $250 each month for every child between 6-17 years old. This provision, unfortunately, ended on December 31, 2021, to the chagrin of many community organizers.[63] Although the IRS made direct deposits into the bank accounts of 80% of the families. I was concerned about the Black families that did not have bank accounts. Many poor people cannot afford the bank fees that are the primary revenue source for banking institutions.

In 2014, I was helping my godfather, Mr. Henry, a retired auto worker, apply for the federal HARP loan program. As I reviewed all of his financial information, I was shocked to see that each month the bank charged him $200 in overdraft fees. "How long has the bank been charging you overdraft fees?" He was 83 years old at the time. "I am not sure, but my savings account is not what it used to be, and I don't know why." Upon, a closer review of his bank statements, I quickly saw how the bank was charging the overdraft fees. Each month, Mr. Henry would pay all his bills by check at the end of each month. His social security and pension payments were directly deposited into his checking account within a few days apart. The bank intentionally changed the order of his banking transactions to maximize the overdraft fees. The larger payments for his mortgage and car loan were processed first, and the ATM transaction and the smaller checks for the utility and insurance bills, phone cable, etc., would then be processed with the overdraft fees. Over a few years, Mr. Henry had paid over $4,000 in overdraft fees that were taken from his savings account.

This was a travesty for a senior citizen on a fixed income. I contacted the bank and spoke to the branch manager to see what could be done. The manager was able to reverse the overdraft fees for the last year which provided some relief. I then worked with Mr. Henry to set up his bill payments to avoid any bank fees. After working with my godfather, I was able to learn first-hand why many people do not have bank accounts. Unfortunately, many new cash transfer apps like PayPal can also charge fees to process specific transactions. The idiom, "the rich get richer, and the poor get poorer" is quite true.

In addition to the CARES Act, the Child Tax Credit increased from $2,000 to $3,600 for each child under six, and an increase from $2,000 to $3,000 for children between the ages of 6 and 17 years old. The cost to the government was approximately $15 billion to support 60 million eligible children out of the $1.9 trillion approved for the American Rescue Plan that was passed in March 2021. The projection was that the new tax credit will reduce child poverty by 50% or five million children in 2021.[64]

What is even more critical to addressing economic stability, is the opportunity for parents to obtain jobs that pay a living wage.

The federal minimum wage is only $8.55 per hour and has not grown with the rate of inflation for the past 30 years. If the minimum wage was adjusted for inflation, it would be $30 per hour. However, one must have a job to afford healthcare. Historically, the Black unemployment rate trend is twice as high as the white unemployment rate. Fifty years ago, the 1970 Black unemployment rate was 8.2 % compared to 4.5% for the white unemployment rate. In October 2021 Black versus white unemployment rate was 7.9% compared to 4.0%.[65]

Black economic stability could be achieved with employment programs, career counseling, and high-quality childcare to ensure that people can not only find but keep jobs. Economic stability will require robust policies to help people pay for food, housing, healthcare, and education as needed to reduce poverty and improve overall health. The goal for economic stability is stable employment with a living wage that allows families to meet the following health challenges:

- Food insecurity
- Problems paying medical bills
- Trouble finding a doctor
- Skip taking medication due to high cost
- Polluted air and water
- Stable housing, transportation
- Safe neighborhood
- Education, job opportunities, stable income
- No access to nutritious foods
- No access to physical exercise

One economic truism is that as the world embraces a new future driven by artificial intelligence, quality education is increasingly more important.

3. Education Access and Quality Pillar

In America, adults with higher levels of education are more likely to be healthier and live longer. Higher education is correlated with more knowledge regarding how to be healthy via food and exercise. However, policies and programs that focus on high-quality educational opportunities for children and adolescents which are important building blocks to reduce healthcare inequity are often absent across the Black community.[66]

The need for good education is essential to good health. However, the United States historically has not supported equitable education for all citizens, separate and unequal, de facto apartheid was the law. For the first two centuries, it was illegal for Black students to attend white schools. In 1954, the landmark Supreme Court decision, Brown vs. Topeka Board of Education, deemed school segregation unconstitutional. The federal government required Southern schools to integrate in the 1960s if they wanted to continue to receive federal funds. The response was the white flight to private and parochial schools.

Over the years, there has been both progress and regression regarding Black education in America. The percentages of Black students in Southern white public schools increased from 23% to a high of 44% from 1968 to 1980.[67] However, the Ronald Reagan and George Bush administrations introduced "School Choice" and "School Excellence" that enabled white schools to re-segregate once again. In 2020, research shows that white students attended the most segregated schools in the country with 73% of white students attending virtually all-white schools. So why is this important? While it is unnecessary for a Black student to sit adjacent to a white student to receive a quality education, it is necessary for a Black student to have access to the same caliber of schools with the same resources. The data demonstrated that public and now some private (called charter) white schools receive more federal, state, and local funding than their Black counterparts. The question is, what is needed for an equitable distribution of public funds? This is the only way to ensure that Black students have access to educational resources. In 2020, the COVID-19 global pandemic had a tremendous impact on schools that were forced to close. The sudden switch to online education required new infrastructure that did not exist for many poorer school districts. Once again, the Black community was hit hard with limited laptops, limited internet access, and limited teaching staff agile enough to pivot from classroom to online learning. The struggle continued as frustrated parents tried to help their children by driving them to Wi-Fi "hot spots" to access the internet. The data have concluded that 2020 was a lost academic year for many Black families. In addition to the Black children having the necessary resources to learn, many did not have access to healthy food with the closure of school and the suspension of the breakfast and lunch programs.

4. Healthcare Access and Quality Pillar

In the United States, HealthCare Access and Quality Healthcare is a challenge for many Black families. The impact of racism on programs that are needed to help them get timely, high-quality healthcare services is astounding. For example, the 2010 Affordable Care Act was a new opportunity for Black people to have access to healthcare insurance and preventative maintenance programs. For the first time, many Black Americans were able to have access to a primary care physician. However, unlike what I experienced as a child with a loving Black healthcare provider, the ability to find a Black physician, Black psychologist, or Black dentist is extremely challenging. Note, although Black people represent

15% of the population, there is huge underrepresentation of Black healthcare professionals at only 5%. As a healthcare consultant, it was extremely rare to consult in primary care offices in which there were any Black physicians, nurses or, even office staff. For example, a pediatric office in a health clinic with an overwhelmingly Black population at 99.5% did not have one Black doctor or nurse. When I did ask the two Black medical assistants who had been with the office for a combined 47 years, why? Their response was that not only had the office never had a Black doctor or a Black nurse in the history of the pediatric practice, but they were treated poorly by the clinician. Although they were trained as medical assistants, their jobs were reclassified as "clerks" and responsible for patient scheduling.

Thus, the predominately, Black patient population had no interaction with the two Black staff members. The medical assistant is responsible for rooming the patient and taking vitals. I asked the elderly white medical director, who was once herself a medical assistant, why the pediatric practice staff did not reflect the population that they served. She became defensive and indicated that the patients were happy with the staff. I conducted a Patient Satisfaction Survey for the practice and the results were disturbing with only 15% of the patients satisfied with the care that they received. Several Black mothers shared in the open comments that they were infuriated when the doctors asked them to leave the examining rooms during the office visit. They later learned that their pre-teen daughters were asked questions about their sexual activity. I was flabbergasted. I confronted the doctors about this, and their response was that it was important for Black girls to be placed on birth control as soon as possible to stop the cycle of teenage pregnancy. Since I could not hire Black physicians, I did create new Standard Operating Procedures to meet patients' needs.

In 2020, it was estimated that 10% of Americans do not have health insurance.[68] For Black Americans, the estimate is that in some counties, that uninsured rate is as high as 25%. For preventative healthcare maintenance, it is essential for people to have a primary care provider, however, this is very unlikely for those without insurance. The other challenge is not being able to afford the healthcare services and medications that are needed to overcome an illness. Federal, state, and local policies are needed to increase insurance coverage rates. This is critical to ensure that more people have access to important healthcare services, like preventive care and treatment for chronic illnesses.

Due to health inequity, Black people may not get the recommended healthcare services including cancer screenings. This may be due to the fact that they either don't have a primary care provider or the providers who offer the screens are several miles away. Well-planned interventions and programs are needed to increase access to healthcare professionals. In addition, better communications between the Black community and healthcare professionals are needed either in person or remotely due to the COVID-19 global pandemic. There are several health issues that affect women more severely than men including breast cancer, death from heart attacks, and osteoarthritis. For Black women, all of these are specific conditions that plague Black women more significantly than white women including diabetes, infertility, and sickle cell disease. When it comes to pregnancy-related issues, Black mothers are known to be more likely to experience traumatic births than other women.[69]

5. Neighborhood and Built Environment Pillar

The neighborhood has a major impact on people's health and well-being. The impact of racism by neighborhood can also be measured by a person's zip code. Yes, in America, healthcare by zip code is parallel to education by zip code in which both can dictate quality and access. When doing healthcare research, many investigators request that the data be available by certain demographics including, age, race, gender, insurance, education, marital status, and zip code. I remember the first time that I asked why zip codes should be captured and was told that the zip code was a good attribute to measure the economic status of a patient when it could not be accessed. When you go to the doctor's office, you are not asked about your income, but you are asked your address which includes your zip code.

America is a truly racially segregated country with white people living in the most segregated areas. Most white Americans are likely to live in a neighborhood that is more than 71% white. [70] The term, "white flight" that originated in the 1940s described the mass exodus of white families from integrated cities to the suburbs. This exodus was facilitated by the federal government and financial institutions that provided federally secured loans to white borrowers and not to Black borrowers. This practice is known as "redlining" due to the maps that identify the Black communities in "red" and white communities in "green." This practice not only prevented Black families from home ownership, but also impeded their ability to obtain wealth. Thus, the racial wealth gap persists.

In 2020, the average white family has 10 times the wealth of the average Black family. It reminds me of a *Pittsburgh Post-Gazette* article regarding the wealth of Americans.[71] It indicated that single Black women have a median wealth of only $5 compared to $42,600 for single white women. The study highlighted this huge disparity during prime working years between the ages of 36 and 49 and concluded that the government must help Black families build wealth in the same way that it helped white Americans. The Homestead Act provided free land to white immigrants, and White veterans received free education from the GI bill.

Discriminatory business loan practices in Black neighborhoods impact access to healthy food and medicine with limited opportunities to buy grocery stores. The number of grocery stores and pharmacies in Black neighborhoods has declined since the 1960s. The "Black Flight" is defined as the migration of Black people from predominately Black neighborhoods to the suburbs after the passage of the 1964 Civil Rights Act. The migration left many Black neighborhoods without a solid Black middle class. The results were the creation of poor Black neighborhoods with few resources. It is quite common for underserved neighborhoods to have "food deserts" which are defined as no local grocery stores with fresh fruits and vegetables. Instead, there may be local corner stores with snacks and processed foods with limited nutritional values. Poor nutrition raises their risk of chronic health conditions like heart disease, diabetes, kidney disease, and obesity. Poor health reduces the quality of life and overall life expectancy.

Unfortunately, simply promoting healthy choices, won't eliminate these and other health disparities. What is the value of a national health campaign that tells the public to eat healthy, if healthy foods are not readily available? Instead, public health organizations and their partners in sectors like education, transportation, and housing must take corrective action to improve the environment. In addition to poor quality food, many poverty-stricken neighborhoods have high rates of violence, unsafe drinking water, poor air quality, and other health and safety risks. Black people with low incomes are more likely to live in places with these risks.

Chapter 4 - Key Points to Remember

1. The 1990s term health equity is when all members of society enjoy a fair and just opportunity to be as healthy as possible. Public health policies and programs centered around the specific needs of communities can promote health equity.[53]

2. The World Health Organization (WHO) states that health inequity is due to human-made systems and structures that privilege certain groups and underserve or actively oppress others. This occurs through the unequal distribution of power and resources.[54]

3. There are five types of health inequities including, racism, sexism, classism, xenophobia, and ableism.

4. The Social Determinants of Health (SDOH) refer to the environments in which people are born, grow, live, work and die. Your health challenges did not begin with your first visit to your doctor's office or being rushed to the emergency room by ambulance. Your healthcare actually began in your mother's womb.

5. There is a racist foundation in the SDOH which includes five pillars: Community & Social Context, Economic Stability, Educations Access & Quality, Healthcare Access & Quality, and Neighborhood Built Environment.

6. In 2020, the overall U.S. poverty rate was 11.4% compared to the Black poverty rate of 19.5% compared to a white poverty rate of only 8.2%.

7. For two centuries, it was illegal for Black students to attend white schools. In 1954, school segregation would legally end with the Brown vs. Topeka Board of Education

supreme court decision. The response to the ruling was white parents enrolling their children in white private and parochial schools. In 2020, research shows that 73% of which children attend virtually all- white schools. The data demonstrates that today, some white private (now called charter) receive more federal, state, and local funding than their Black counterparts.

8. In 2020, it was estimated that 10% of Americans do not have health insurance and for Black Americans, the estimate may be as high as 25% in some counties. This results in limited healthcare access and poorer health outcomes.

9. In American healthcare, status can be determined by zip code. Black neighborhoods do not receive the same amount of government or economic support for intergenerational wealth building. In the 1940s, the white flight to the suburbs was enabled by federally secured home loans to white borrowers. The practice was known as "redlining" due to maps that identified Black communities in "red" and white communities in "green."

10. Black people with low incomes as much as 25% are more likely to live in neighborhoods with no grocery stores, poor quality schools, no hospitals, higher rates of violence, unsafe drinking water, poor air quality, and other health and safety risks.

CHAPTER 5:
UNDERSTANDING THE IMPACT OF RACISM IN HEALTHCARE – HEALTH DISPARITIES

In the United States, examples of health disparities have become more apparent with the COVID-19 global pandemic. March 2021 Data showed that nationwide, Black people have died from COVID-19 at 1.4 times the rate of white people which is the highest for all racial categories. At least 73,462 Black lives have been lost due to COVID-19. However, many states are not reporting death by race, thus the actual number is unknown.

In engineering, there is a saying adopted from Lord Kelvin, *"If you cannot measure it, you cannot improve it."* [72] Thus, the data on health disparities are needed and tell a tragic story. As an engineer and healthcare consultant, my role is to analyze data and identify solutions that provide measurable improvement.

To adequately measure if the health system is equitable, health institutions collect data on health outcomes and quantify the disparities. The Centers for Disease Control and Prevention (CDC) identifies health disparities as follows:

> "The preventable differences in the burden of disease, injury, violence, or opportunities to achieve optimal health that are experienced by socially disadvantaged populations." [73]

For example, in the medical community, studies have demonstrated that medical professionals do not treat patients the same. A 2020 study showed that there are racial disparities that are very apparent regarding pain treatment.[74] The studies show that Black patients are significantly less likely to be prescribed pain medication and that they generally receive lower doses of it. One possible reason for this, supported by existing studies, is that white people believe Black people experience less pain.

The United States is home to stark and persistent racial disparities in health coverage, chronic health conditions, mental health, and mortality. These disparities are not a result of individual or group behavior but decades of systematic inequality in American economic, housing, and health care systems.

This fact sheet sheds light on some of the most persistent inequities facing African Americans or Black Americans, Hispanic Americans or Latinx Americans, Asian Americans, Native Hawaiian or other Pacific Islander Americans, and American Indians or Alaska Natives. Alleviating health disparities will require a deliberate and sustained effort to address social determinants of health, such as poverty, segregation, environmental degradation, and racial discrimination.

The 2019 health disparities for Black, Hispanic, and White Americans are listed in Table 9.[75]

Table 9.

American Health Disparities by Race

	American Health Disparity Description	Black Americans	Hispanic Americans	White Americans
Health Coverage	Uninsured (all ages)	10.6%	16.1%	5.9%
	Uninsured < 65 years old	12.1%	20.1%	8.0%
	Health coverage	89.4%	83.9%	93.7%
	Medicaid Beneficiary	37.0%	32.0%	19.0%
Chronic Health Conditions	Fair or Poor Health	13.8%	10.0%	8.3%
	Obesity (Adults)*	38.0%	34.9%	31.0%
	Hypertension (Adults)*	32.2%	23.7%	23.9%
	Diabetes (Diagnosed Adults)*	13.1%	13.2%	8.6%
	Chronic Kidney Disease	16.0%	11.9%	15.7%
Mortality	Cancer Mortality Rate (per 100,000)	171.0	105.6	151.4
	Infant Mortality Rate (per 100,000)	10.8	5.6	4.5
	Maternal Mortality Rate (per 100,000)	37.1	11.8	14.7
	2019 Life Expectancy (years)	74.7	81.8	78.8

An American human tragedy is the plight of Black mothers and families who suffer an unimaginable loss due to infant mortality. In 2018, Black infant mortality was 2.3 times that rate of whites, and the top five leading causes of death were the following:

1. Low-Birthweight
2. Congenital malformations
3. Maternal complications
4. Sudden Infant Death Syndrome (SIDS)
5. Accidents (unintentional injuries)

There is one attribute that is not listed in the statistics, and that is the stress of being Black in America. The constant stress of being a member of a group that is both marginalized and devalued can be extremely debilitating, not to mention mentally exhausting. This condition is only compounded for Black women during pregnancy. I can recall the countless number of times friends and family united to support a recent new mom in the loss of her infant son or daughter due to the death. A root cause analysis yielded systemic racism as the culprit. The myriad stories of how they were disrespected during their doctor's appointments including snide comments about their weight or eating habits. The unnecessary stress at their jobs and having to negotiate time away to attend their doctors' appointments. In addition, the constant worry about whether or not they would even have a job if they did not return to work shortly after giving birth. The fact is that Black men and women have higher unemployment rates, lower wages, and lower wealth making it nearly impossible to take advantage of unpaid medical leave to support an ill family member or a newborn.

When I worked at a Swedish pharmaceutical company, I learned about how the Swedish labor union supported both maternity and paternity leave. Both the new mom and new dad received one year of paid maternity and paid paternity leave that could be taken consecutively, thus giving two full years of parental leave. Research studies indicate that the primary benefits of paid parental leave not only allow time away from work to allow mothers to recover from childbirth but also to care for a newborn. Other striking benefits are the reduction in infant mortality and improved maternal mental health. In America, Black parents are not afforded paid parental leave like Swedish parents. Also, in Sweden, as in other countries, their rate of death is much lower than Americans.

The leading causes of U. S. deaths are shown in Table 10 below.[76]

Table 10.
Top 5 Leading Causes of Death in the U. S.

Rank	Cause	Number of Deaths/Year
1	Heart Disease	655,381
2	Cancer	599,274
3	COVID-19	299,445*
4	Medical Errors	251,000
5	Accidents - unintentional injuries	167,127

**Based on data retrieved at 1:00 PM on 12.14.20 from Johns Hopkins Coronavirus Resource Center*

https://www.sokolovelaw.com/blog/covid-19-is-3rd-leading-cause-of-death-in-the-u-s/

What are Hospital Medical Errors?

Unfortunately, medical errors in American Hospitals are ubiquitous and account for over 250,000 deaths per year. Table 10 shows the top five leading causes of death in the United States. Thus, in 2020, Medical Errors are the fourth leading cause of death after COVID-19.[77]

When it comes to medical errors, the most common mistakes made by doctors that lead to death include:

- Misdiagnosis
- Delayed diagnosis
- Medication error
- Infection
- Misuse of antibiotics
- Premature patient discharge

Identified by the U.S. Department of Health and Human Services (HHS) as "root causes" of medical-error-related deaths, the following factors often lead to errors committed by medical professionals: [77]

- **Communication problems:** Miscommunication between hospital staff, between hospital divisions, or between hospitals.

- **Inadequate information flow:** Necessary information may not follow the patient upon transfer to another service or discharge.

- **Human error:** Failures in following policies, guidelines, protocols, and processes, including poor documentation and labeling of samples and specimens.

- **Patient-related issues:** Wrong patient identification, partial or incomplete patient assessment, and failure to obtain consent.

- **Staffing patterns and workflow:** Problems resulting from overworked and tired healthcare workers, poor supervision, and inadequate staffing.

- **Technological failures:** Medical device failures, including poorly designed medical devices or equipment and/or improper medical device handling or implantation.

- **Inadequate policies and procedures:** Problems in the process of care are often traced to poorly documented, non-existent, or clinically inadequate procedures.

Given the various circumstances that can produce medical errors, tracking them can be exceedingly difficult. While there certainly needs to be increased transparency on the part of doctors and hospitals, the system itself needs updating to meet the demands of the 21st century.

Unfortunately, as a healthcare consultant, I have worked on projects that were a response to Medical Errors. In 2017, I worked on an Ambulatory Infusion Center FMEA project. The hospital leaders labeled the infusion center as the most dangerous place in the hospital due to many medical errors that resulted in patient harm in a one-year period. One of the errors resulted in the patient being given the wrong blood product during a medical infusion. I worked with the Infusion Leader and Staff and conducted a failure mode and effects analysis (FMEA).

What is FMEA?

Failure Mode and Effects Analysis (FMEA) is a structured way to identify and address potential problems, or failures and their resulting effects on the system or process before an adverse event occurs. In comparison, Root Cause Analysis (RCA) is a structured way to address problems after they occur.

As the consultant, I led the team to identify all the current state process steps from the time the Infusion Center appointment was scheduled to the time that the patient completed their appointment. The RCA showed myriad reasons for the medical errors. However, the main cause was that the Infusion Center did not have nursing assignments. The results showed that one patient could have as many as five nurses during her appointment. This was in contrast to other infusion centers that would have only one nurse assigned to the patients, which is the standard for hospital patients.

The serious consequence of having multiple nurses monitoring multiple patients was that medical errors could occur. In the case of the administration of the wrong blood product was as follows: the patient had arrived for a blood transfusion. In this process, the nurse has to check the patient's wristband, the blood product identification, and the physician's order. This was done with the first bag of blood. The first nurse did the proper identification and hung the blood bag on the IV pole. The patient was then monitored to ensure that there were no adverse reactions. The nurse is then required to initial her check on the monitoring log that is on the patient's chart. During the first hour, two different nurses had monitored the patient. When it was time for the second bag, a third nurse decided to administer the second bag which was on the table near the patient. The third nurse assumed that the double patient identification had been done on all of the blood bags for the patients and hung the blood bag. This was the wrong blood.

Once the patient began receiving the product, per the Event Report, the adverse reaction was immediate. The patient was rushed to the emergency room, which was down a long corridor. The patient received emergency care and recovered. The FMEA found that in addition to no nursing assignments, poor communication, and poor training were also root causes. As the healthcare consultant, my goal was to have the nursing manager and staff identify solutions that everyone would support. Once the results of the FMEA were reviewed, the next step was to identify solutions to reduce the risk of medical errors. In addition, I facilitated multiple team-building workshops to help the small staff improve team performance.

The results were impressive. The Ambulatory Infusion Center was redesigned and nursing assignments were implemented. The nursing assignments allowed the nurses to be dedicated to their patients exclusively from arrival to departure. A daily huddle was launched to help with communication and problem-solving. One of the daily topics was "Barriers for the Day." For example, if there was an "Add-On,"defined as a patient that was added to the schedule on the same day, the team was able to have a brief discussion on which nurse should take that assignment. This was a better method than the nurse manager deciding which nurse would take the assignment. Another change was a new buddy system that allowed each nurse to have a buddy that would cover their assignment during bathroom and lunch breaks. Both the daily huddle and buddy system were well received and improved team performance. The number of medical errors was reduced to zero after the launch of the redesign.

Another devastating medical mistake involved my husband. In 2005, my husband was rushed to the hospital after he passed out after playing tennis in 100 degress-F heat. I witnessed my husband convulsing as his eyes rolled back in his head before he blacked out. Luckily, this was a tournament that required that a nurse be available. I yelled for the nurse. She came over and asked me what happened. "My husband had just won his match and he sat down. He then put his head down and I asked him if he was okay. He began convulsing and his eyes rolled back." The nurse asked for ice. The goal was to cool my husband down because he was suffering from dehydration. The paramedics arrived and we went to the nearest hospital. It was a Saturday and there was the weekend staff.

What is Weekend Staff?

Although the emergency room is opened 24 hours per day, 7 days per week, that does not mean that the ancillary support staff is available including laboratories, therapists, imaging, and more. It is possible that due to weekend staff shortages, many of the tests that a patient might need, would not be available until Monday.

The EMT (Emergency Management Technician) had contacted the emergency room from the ambulance. Upon arrival, my husband and I were told that due to weekend staff, we would have to wait until Monday for laboratory tests. He was admitted to the hospital as a precaution. Once we arrived at his room, my husband insisted that he was okay. He wanted to go home. I wanted answers to understand why he blacked out.

On Monday, the lab tests that were ordered were administered. The results were returned and showed possible heart issues may be the cause of my husband's collapse. We were shocked. My husband was healthy and played multiple supports including tennis and basketball. I called my husband's primary care physician and he recommended that we have a consult with one of his trusted colleagues, a cardiologist. Both were African Americans and showed true concern for my husband's health. Additional tests were done and my husband's heart was fine. His syncope, i.e., black out was due to severe dehydration.

However, the following day, my husband called me in distress. It was around 7:00 am, and he told me that a team of white coats were in his room and wanted to discuss his pacemaker. He stated that he was not getting a pacemaker. I went to the hospital and asked to speak to the surgeon. The surgeon came to the room and essentially restated what he told my husband. I then asked an important question, "Who ordered the pacemaker." He gave the name of the cardiologist, who we did not recognize. It was then I asked, "Do you have the right Richard Johnson?" My husband with the very common names of both Richard and Johnson. We were told that there were over 100 patients with the same name. That was the issue. A medical error, because a "unique identifier" for patients with common names had not been identified. When patients have a common name, a "unique identifier" is required to make sure that this is the correct patient. Typically, it is the birthday.

This was a simple medical error that could have been easily avoided by checking the birthdates of the pacemaker surgical order and my husband's information. I am thankful that my husband was able to find his voice and tell the surgical team that they had the wrong Richard Johnson.

The health disparities of Black and white Americans continue today as they did during enslavement. To address what is wrong today, an understanding of the inequities of the past is imperative. Only then can we begin to dismantle the structural racism that is replete within the American system. Knowledge of the history of racism in healthcare is necessary to explore and identify the underlying mechanisms to understand how racism revives itself to continue to produce health disparities and ways to interrupt it.

PART 2

MY HEALTHCARE NIGHTMARE – LUCKY TO BE ALIVE

CHAPTER 6: MY INITIAL EMERGENCY ROOM VISITS

My Healthcare Emergencies

It was August 1986, and I was rushed to the hospital. I had been throwing up for a few days and I did not know what was happening to my otherwise healthy body. The symptoms included vomiting and sharp lower abdominal pains. My final diagnosis was gall bladder disease, and I needed a cholecystectomy. My gall bladder had to be removed. The surgeon assured me and my mother that the gall bladder was essentially a reservoir that held bile that was released after eating a fat-rich diet. Wow! I then mentally inventoried my recent meals. Yes! It had to have been the bologna sandwich with extra cheese that I ate as I travelled by car from South Carolina to Pennsylvania. I was not sure what to think about the need for surgery. I felt that a second opinion was warranted, however, the pain was overwhelming.

The surgery was scheduled by the emergency surgery team. Ironically, it was the same surgical group that had also left me disfigured after my botched breast surgery the prior year. That is another sad story about healthcare racism. Needless to say, I was extremely nervous. The surgery was supposedly simple. A diagonal incision to extricate the diseased gall bladder was supposedly routine. However, what should have been routine, was not the case.

My mom was in my room when the surgeon arrived shortly after my surgery. He had a worried look on his face. He informed us that the surgery did not go as planned. He then began to draw a diagram on the hospital room whiteboard. He spoke as he drew the diagram. "The cystic bile ducts that are used to transfer bile to the stomach to help with food digestion were blocked by a gallstone," he explained.

The stone was about the size of a small pea, approximately a quarter inch in diameter. The blocked cystic bile duct was the source of my severe pain. I then asked, "Why wasn't the stone removed first and why can't it be removed now?" His response was strange. "Unfortunately, the stone could not be removed." So, he then explained that I had to return to the operating room and a tube will be inserted in the cystic bile duct and extend outside of my body. The tube would be attached to a bile bag which would be strapped to my leg. I would have to empty the bag throughout the day. The tube will allow scar tissue to be formed around the tube and create a tunnel. After six weeks, a small catheter will be inserted into the newly formed tunnel to retrieve the stone.

My mind was racing. How did this happen? Wasn't there a process to see if the stone that caused the problem was removed upon removing my gall bladder? I did not have the voice to request better quality care. So, I relented. My mom relented, and I went home with a bile bag attached to my leg. In the required time period, I returned to the hospital, and I was able to watch the procedure as the stone was removed. I prayed to God that I would never experience this horrific malpractice again but to my disappointment that was not the case. In 2019, it was déjà vu.

March 17, 2019, Sunday Afternoon

On March 17, 2019, I was experiencing abdominal pain that was eerily similar to my gall bladder symptoms in 1986. However, this time as a healthcare consultant, I reviewed my previous healthcare encounters with a different lens. What has been common in all of my hospital and surgical encounters were the following:

- 100% of my physicians were white
- 100% of my surgeons were white
- Nearly 100% of my nurses were white
- 100% of the hospital medical leaders were white

What was different this time was that my husband was my advocate instead of my mother. Needless to say, the pain was excruciating, and I was vomiting incessantly. I was in a full emergency that required immediate medical attention.

My husband took me to the emergency room near our home. It was a free-standing facility which is different from a hospital that has an operating room and in-patient beds. So, if I needed to have surgery, I would have to be transferred to a hospital for urgent emergency care services. My husband and I arrived at the nearest ER in the early afternoon. The place was not crowded, and I counted four other patients in the waiting area. I was triaged immediately which was the first step of our emergency room visit where my medical problem was assessed and assigned an Emergency Severity Index (ESI) level. In my case, a registered triage nurse dealt with me, and I was assessed as a level 4. I was too ill to fight my level assignment of only a level 4 instead of level 2 which means life-threatening. In my head, I am thinking *"My condition was deemed semi-urgent and not urgent?"* I was asked to return to the waiting room after my registration. I then waited for an hour to be sent to an examination room.

What I have learned as a healthcare consultant is that triage is an important step that dictates what will happen next. Thus, the triage nurse has a lot of power and can decide which patients would receive immediate attention and which patients would have to wait. In my case, there were two options, in which I was assigned option 2.

1. Patient is taken to an exam room. If all rooms are full, that person will be next in line for a room based on the severity of their condition.

2. Patient is asked to return to the waiting room and wait to be called.

As I was waiting to be called to the examination room, a thousand thoughts raced through my mind. Most healthcare systems can have myriad emergency examination rooms that service many patients 24 hours per day. Unfortunately, you can have an extremely long wait if your triage assessment deems that your symptoms are not a level 1 or level 2. An interesting caveat is that depending on your insurance coverage, and if your illness is not an emergency, your insurance provider may recommend that you go to an urgent care center or schedule an appointment with your primary care physician. Unsurprisingly, the main objective is for the insurance company to save money due to the costs of emergency care, and to that end, the patient will have a higher co-pay for the emergency room visit.

Again, after the triage nurse completed her assessment, my husband and I returned to the Emergency Room waiting area due to my lower emergency severity index or ESI score. Remember, a level 4, is considered urgent but not l life-threatening. After an hour, we went to the examination room where a physician completed a physical exam, which is to evaluate your symptoms and medical history along with a physical exam. The emergency room doctor will:

1. Check your vital signs including blood pressure, and temperature.
2. Listen to your belly with a stethoscope. Appendicitis may reduce the normal sounds made by the colon.
3. Touch or press certain places on your belly. The way it feels in different spots can be a sign of appendicitis.
4. Perform a rectal exam, as in some cases appendicitis can cause rectal pain.
5. Perform a pelvic exam on women of childbearing age. Your doctor will examine the female reproductive organs to rule out conditions that mimic appendicitis.

Serendipity will prove to be salient during my medical emergency. I will tell you how: in 2014, I was the consultant responsible for creating a new Acute Appendicitis Surgical Care Plan. To prepare, I conducted extensive research on acute appendicitis to determine the opportunities to improve clinical outcomes. I learned that appendicitis is a common condition.

Appendicitis is an inflammation of a small pouch in the colon called the appendix that is the size of your pinkie finger. The treatment is for a surgeon to remove the appendix by performing an appendectomy. I learned that the most classic symptom of appendicitis is severe pain in the right lower abdominal area. However, although this is a major symptom, many other problems can cause the same type of pain. Thereby, it is important for the emergency doctor to find the cause of your symptoms before recommending surgery. Also, the patient can't diagnose if they have appendicitis by themselves. I also learned that not everyone has the same kind of abdominal pain or the same symptoms during appendicitis. For example, the pain may not be as severe for every patient, or you may have pain in a different abdominal area along with a fever, or nausea, and vomiting.

After an exam, your doctor will want to do some lab tests to confirm acute appendicitis. The results will show problems that typically occur with appendicitis. Your doctor will also use the test results to rule out other causes of your symptoms. This helps your doctor make the best treatment decisions for you. Other tests will include:

1. Blood tests. A complete blood count (CBC) shows inflammation or infection in the body. A chemistry panel reveals dehydration and fluid and electrolyte imbalances.

2. Pregnancy test - Some problems of pregnancy, such as morning sickness or a miscarriage, can appear like appendicitis. Doctors also use this test to make sure they use medications that are safe during pregnancy.

3. Urine test - A urinalysis can help show a bladder infection, kidney stone, or poor kidney function. It also helps your doctor choose medications that are safe for your kidneys.

4. Your doctor will also likely order one or more of the following noninvasive imaging tests if you have signs of appendicitis such as a CT scan which creates an X-ray-based image of your belly area. They help diagnose appendicitis or find other reasons for your symptoms. Your doctor can see much more detail with a CT scan compared to a regular X-ray or ultrasound.

It is imperative for the doctor to make the correct diagnosis since several other conditions can cause low abdominal pain including uterine fibroids, pancreatitis, and other types of intestinal inflammation. The emergency doctor will need to do a thorough evaluation to find the cause of your symptoms.

After receiving the lab and CT scan results, my husband and I are informed of my diagnosis. I was informed that I have acute appendicitis and emergency surgery is needed. It had now been seven hours since our arrival at the Emergency Room. However, we would have to travel to the hospital. We arrive at the hospital at 11 pm. It was now 8 hours since my ER arrival. I am immediately admitted to the hospital to a nursing unit and asked to completely undress and put on a hospital gown in preparation for my surgery. Again, per my work as a healthcare consultant, I had led the team that created the *Acute Appendicitis Surgical Care Plan* in 2014. That plan required that a patient diagnosed with acute appendicitis has 8 hours to get to the operating room.

The surgeon entered my hospital room. and I recognized him immediately. He was actually on the *Acute Appendicitis Surgical Care Plan* team. I finally had an opportunity to talk to the surgeon about my appendectomy. He informed us that there is an alternative to the traditional appendectomy. The new protocol is called, "conservative management." I was clueless. During the project team meeting when we created the Acute Appendicitis Surgical Care Plan, the only treatment was an appendectomy.

March 18, 2019, Monday, 1:00 am

Unfortunately, as it was 1:00 am on a Monday, I was in no condition to argue about the merits of conservative management or whether or not I was a good candidate for this new protocol.

I later did some research and found the following in the article, "Surgery for appendicitis: is it necessary?" Author Rodney Mason, concludes the following:

> "Appendectomy for acute appendicitis is an effective, universally accepted procedure performed more than 300,000 times annually in the United States. It is generally believed that appendicitis progresses invariably from early inflammation to later gangrene and perforation, and that appendectomy is required for surgical source control. Although non-operative management with antibiotics of uncomplicated diverticulitis, salpingitis, and neonatal enterocolitis is now established, the non-operative management of appendicitis remains largely unexplored. Appendectomy may not be necessary for the majority of patients with acute uncomplicated appendicitis, as many patients resolve spontaneously and others may be treatable with antibiotics alone. However, the supporting documentation is scant and of poor quality." [78]

Due to the poor quality of conservation management for acute appendicitis research, the gold standard for acute appendicitis is an appendectomy.

At that time, I was in debilitating pain and I desperately wanted it to stop. I had never heard of conservative management, and since I knew the surgeon, I wanted to trust his opinion. However, my gut was telling me that this was a grave mistake. My head was spinning from the conflicting information and advice. I had acute appendicitis, and instead of doing surgery, I was placed on antibiotics instead of being in the operating room awaiting life-saving surgery. It was 2:00 am, so I told my husband to go home and get some sleep. I began to pray and asked God to watch over me. The medications finally kicked in and I drifted off to sleep. Around 6:00 am, I heard a voice, "Dr. Johnson. Are you awake?" The physician doing the rounds introduced the members of the Patient-Centered Rounds (PCR) team which is a practice in which the physician, bedside nurse, case manager, and specialists enter the room and talk to the patient. The patient is the "center" of the communication. As a healthcare consultant, I did observations on PCRs and was well aware of the practice. Unfortunately, I was barely awake and was not an active participant in the rounding experience.

Ideally, the PCR was an opportunity for me to learn about my plan of care (POC) and my discharge date (DC) and ask questions. The physician led the discussion. As my case summary was reviewed, I was disoriented due to the medication and not able to clearly articulate my thoughts. I remembered them telling me that I will be discharged the following day, and prescribed a ten-day antibiotic regimen. I asked about the surgery. and again, I was told that I was on a "conservative management" protocol. At the time, I did not know the criteria for "conservative management." I was literally dazed and confused. They ended the round with their discharge plan.

A safe discharge from the hospital requires that the following takes place:

- **Evaluation** of the patient by qualified personnel.
- **Discussion** with the patient or his representative.
- **Planning** for homecoming or transfer to another care facility.
- **Determining** whether caregiver training or other support is needed.
- **Referrals** to a home care agency and/or appropriate support organizations in the community.
- **Arranging** for follow-up appointments or tests.

March 19, 2019, Tuesday morning, 7:00 am

I was discharged the following Tuesday at 7:00 am with a physician's order. I thought to myself, *"Is this a safe discharge?"* I should have had an appendectomy which was the standard treatment for my diagnosis. I was not asked if I had someone home for support and whether or not I could take care of myself. I said to myself, this is not a safe discharge. However, I failed to voice my concerns.

So, I was being discharged with acute appendicitis with instructions comprising a ten-day regimen of the antibiotic, Augmentin (Amoxicillin and Clavulante), and Tylenol for pain. I was also instructed to follow up with my primary care physician (PCP). During my hospital stay, I was on intravenous medication, including the opioid, oxycodone, and the antibiotic, Zosyn. However, my prescription was only for Augmentin. Instead of being prescribed a pill form of opioid for pain, I was told that I can take Tylenol if I continue to have pain or a fever. A well-known healthcare fact is that Black patients are told that their pain is not serious based on a legacy of racist beliefs that Black people do not feel pain. I was in severe pain and was only told to take Tylenol.

My husband arrived in the hospital room to take me home. The nurse reviewed the discharge instructions with the two of us and asked us if we had any questions. As a healthcare consultant, I worked with a hospital to create the patient discharge question list below:

1. What was the final diagnosis?
2. Is a follow-up appointment needed?
3. What medications have been prescribed?
4. What should I do when I get home?
5. Do I need to have someone with me at home?
6. When can I return to work?

7. Who do I call if my pain gets worse?
8. What is the likelihood that I will be readmitted?

Unfortunately, I lacked the mental acuity to ask the appropriate questions during my discharge. I was discharged with "acute appendicitis" and told that I would have surgery after my appendix "calmed down." What exactly did that mean? I was fully stressed and wondering why I was treated with no regard for my health and safety.

My husband was worried and concerned. He shared a story with me that I had not heard during the twenty-two years of our beloved union. His sister went to the hospital emergency room with abdominal pain and was diagnosed with acute appendicitis and sent home with antibiotics. Her appendix ruptured and she died. He was fearful that I would have the same outcome. I then understood his numbness and his disconnect during my emergency room visit because, for him, this was déjà vu.

CHAPTER 7: FIGHTING FOR QUALITY HEALTHCARE TO SAVE MY LIFE

After I arrived home from my horrific discharge from the hospital without an appendectomy, which is the gold standard treatment for acute appendicitis, I immediately called my primary care physician and scheduled an appointment. She was out of the office attending a conference. My appointment was for March 28, 2019, which was within my 10-day protocol for Augmentin and Tylenol. I had been seeing the same primary care physician for over twenty years. She is originally from Turkey and came to the United States as a teenager. We have a good relationship and she knew me very well. When I arrived at her office, I was not feeling well at all. She entered the exam room, took one look at me, and said, "You look horrible." I remember that I responded, "I feel horrible." She stated that she had reviewed my CT scan and that I needed an emergency appendectomy. She stated that she did not understand why my appendix was not removed when I went to the emergency room. She gave me the name of a surgeon (who I will call, Dr. Williams) who worked at a different hospital. She told me to call him immediately to schedule my emergency appendectomy. She added that I needed to sue the hospital that refused to do my surgery. "Your life is at risk."

As soon as I returned home, I called the recommended surgeon and was surprised that he actually answered the phone. He stated that my PCP had shared my CT scans and that he was familiar with my case. He then stated something that surprised me. "Your PCP is overreacting. Your surgery can be done in a few weeks." I asked him if I was at risk of my appendix rupturing. He assured me that I should continue the "conservative management" treatment. He stated that he would like to see me in 4 days. for an examination after which he would schedule the appendectomy, which would be performed laparoscopically. It was Thursday and he wanted me to wait until the following Tuesday to see him and then he would then schedule my appendectomy. It was late in the evening and I was in shock that another surgeon did not see my acute appendicitis as life-threatening.

March 29, 2019, Friday, 9:00 am

I called my primary care physician who was with a patient. When she returned my phone call, I relayed the disturbing conversation with Dr. Williams. "Dr. Williams stated that you are overreacting, and he refused to do an emergency appendectomy (by default he agreed with the previous surgeons)." My PCP was livid. She told me to stop taking the Tylenol and antibiotics and go to the emergency room immediately and demand the surgery. I called my husband and explained what happened and told him I needed him to come home.

By the time my husband returned home, I had a high fever and chills. This time my husband took me to the hospital emergency room straight away.

I went through triage and due to my recent discharge, I was immediately taken to an exam room. As I undressed, I begged my husband to not let me leave the hospital without the appendectomy. He agreed. The ER physician assistant entered the room and stated that I needed to have another CT scan. I told them that the antibiotic was not working and that my PCP stated that I needed an emergency appendectomy. He expressed his concern that I was back in the emergency room so soon after the discharge. He asked me to evaluate my pain level on a scale of 1 to 10. I told him that it was an 11. I explained to him that I had a fever, chills, and night sweats. He took notes during the examination. The next step was for me to get another CT scan.

March 29, 2019, Friday, 2:30 pm

I was finally getting my second CT scan. I began reflecting on how I got to my tragic state. My ruminations were quite illuminating as outlined below:

"On March 17, 2019, I went to the Emergency Room and was diagnosed with acute appendicitis. I was denied the routine appendectomy via laparoscopic surgery. I remember watching TV and it was reported that the CBS news anchor Norah O'Donnell was on a skiing trip and was rushed to the hospital. She was diagnosed with acute appendicitis and had an emergency appendectomy via laparoscopic surgery. They expected her to return to the airways in a couple of weeks.

She was a white female TV personality, and her acute appendicitis experience was much different than mine. I was back in the emergency room after being discharged with prescribed antibiotics and Tylenol for acute appendicitis. It was apparent that the antibiotics were not working. I had a fever, and chills and was in extreme pain. I questioned why I was being treated with this "conservative management" protocol instead of having an appendectomy. Why didn't

Norah O'Donnell get sent home with antibiotics and Tylenol? I began fretting that I may end up like my sister-in-law whom I never met because she was sent home with acute appendicitis, her appendix ruptured, and she died. I prayed for God's favor and protection."

The patient escort arrived in the room to transport me to the CT department for the CT scan. The escort was a young Black woman with a small frame. My husband joked with her as she moved me and the stretcher around several tight corners. She was petite but strong and navigated the stretcher around each corner like a pro. As we traversed several corridors, I kept praying to God to heal my mind, body, and spirit. I was trying my best to be brave, but my body was letting me know that I was not well.

Upon arrival at the CT scan room, we met the technician and she asked me if I was able to get on the CT scan table. Despite being in so much pain, I still managed to get on the table. The CT scan is a long machine with a small circular opening. Once inside, the scanning commenced and I began to pray. I knew that I was desperately ill and needed an appendectomy. After the scan, I was escorted back to the emergency room by stretcher.

March 29, 2019, Friday, 9:00 am - 5:45 pm

A team of "White Coats" arrived in my examination room. I felt like Dorothy at end of *The Wizard of Oz* when there was a group of people surrounding her when she awakened from her dream of the Land of Oz. However, unlike Dorothy, I was very much awake. This was not a dream. So, who were the "White Coats?" They all introduced themselves: a surgeon, a surgical resident, an infection specialist, a physician assistant, and an ER nurse. The surgeon was a small white woman with short hair. I immediately recognized her from a seminar that I recently attended.

She stated that upon review of my CT scan, she did not recommend that I have the appendectomy.

She then added, "We were all in the CT scan room and we watched you get on the table. You were able to move very well so you can't be in that much pain." I was in shock when she admitted that I was being watched during my CT scan. The audacity! Or how disrespectful! I was furious that she concluded that I am not in pain.

My heart sank as I responded, "It is obvious to me that I need an appendectomy and that it should have been done during my last hospital visit, so what has changed?" She had the computer on wheels (COW) and asked the surgical resident to pull up my CT scan. She explained that I had a new problem. My colon was now inflamed along with my appendix. She stated that if she removed my appendix, there was no healthy tissue to suture upon removal of my appendix. She also explained that there was a rim of what she described as phlegm in my stomach that was also a problem.

My mind was racing. She then asked, "Do you want to live the rest of your life with a colostomy bag? Because that would be the surgical outcome." I felt that she was definitely threatening me. She stated that my colon would heal and that I could have the appendectomy in four weeks. I really had no time to process what she just shared with me and my husband.

The next person to speak was an older white male with glasses and white hair. He stated that he was an infection specialist and had reviewed my case. He then stated, "I think that I know what happened to you and why your body is not responding to the antibiotic. During your last hospital visit, you were given Zosyn, a powerful IV antibiotic for abdominal infections. However, you were prescribed Amoxycillin at discharge because Zosyn can only be administered intravenously. The Amoxycillin is not a strong antibiotic compared to Zosyn." He then went on to state that the new care plan was for me to be admitted to the hospital to get a Peripherally Inserted Central Catheter (PICC) line. This will allow me to get Zosyn intravenously. My immediate thought is "No." I do not want to increase my risk for additional infection by getting a permanent tube placed in a vein in my arm. The surgeon chimed in. "The PICC line can stay in your arm for 4 weeks, and then you will have the appendectomy. My head was swirling ... this was not happening to me. I really did not have time to fully process the information that was just shared.

What Next?

The physician assistant who recommended that I have surgery was still in the room. I immediately asked him his opinion and he agreed that surgery would be the best option and said that however, he is not a surgeon.

This was now the "third surgeon" to refuse to perform my appendectomy. I discussed the new care plan with my husband. He simply says, "Maybe you should wait for the surgery, you don't want to get a colostomy and need an ostomy bag?" In my mind, I am thinking that a colostomy may be better than dying. However, I do not say that to my husband who is already thinking that I may die like his beloved sister. I reluctantly agree to be admitted. "Okay. I will get the PICC line and wait for the appendectomy."

March 30, 2019, Saturday, 9:00 am – Getting a PICC Line

After being admitted to the hospital for a second time, I was scheduled for the PICC line insertion the next day, which was Saturday. As I was being transported to the X-Ray room of the Infusion Department, I felt my nerves on edge. While I was in my hospital room, I quickly researched the PICC line insertion procedures on my laptop. The technician asked me if I wanted to watch, and I answered "yes." As a consultant, I had conducted endless observations in operating rooms, surgery centers, and recently the infusion center, and then I observed my own procedure. How interesting was that? As I watched the X-ray screen, I could see the small catheter that was inserted into my left inner arm, traveling up my arm, down my chest, and stopping right above my heart. I was simultaneously amazed and frightened! The risk for infection had now increased tremendously with a new catheter in my body. Upon completion, the technician placed a red band on my wrist that had information regarding my arm size and the placement of the catheter, which will prove to be extremely important later.

The technician called the patient escort and I returned to my room. I tried my best to rest but to no avail. My catheter was the entry point for my IV fluids and I was told that it was imperative I avoid contracting an infection at all costs. Since the catheter was near my heart, the risk of death was extremely high. I was alone and I did not want to worry my family or friends about my second hospitalization. My husband arrived later in the afternoon. I was losing weight due to the acute appendicitis and I was concerned that I was not getting better. I told him that at that point, I just wanted to go home. He looked concerned, but told me to hang in there.

March 31, 2019, Sunday, 10:00 am

The only change to the routine was a visit by the infusion nurse whose role was to check my PICC line and ensure that there were no infections. As she examined my arm, she expressed concern.

She said, "Your arm looks swollen and there is redness at the site. You may have an infection. You need to go to X-Ray to make sure that your PICC line is placed properly."

Feeling emotional and in denial, I responded, "My arm is not swollen."

She disagreed and informed another nurse that I needed to go to the infusion department. I was now alarmed! *"If I have an infection, what will happen to me?"* I had so many unanswered questions that remained in my mind.

Upon my return to the infusion X-Ray room, I was seen by a different technician. She performed the X-Ray to confirm the catheter placement. She checked my red wristband and looked befuddled. I asked her if everything was okay. She said, "No. Your original measurements are incorrect." The first technician had incorrectly recorded my arm diameter. My arm was not swollen. The emergency X-Ray showed that all was well and that there was a medical error. I breathed a sigh of relief. My anxiety was real but unnecessary. So, after being a victim of a medical error, I contacted the infusion department manager and recommended that they create a new double measurement confirmation method to be implemented. This will ensure that the correct PICC measurements are properly recorded. My recommendation was well received and immediately implemented for safety. I was blessed that my medical error resulted in "over processing" which simply means that extra work had to be performed due to the wrong arm measurement.

Learning How to Administer At-Home IV Infusions

Upon my second hospital discharge, my husband and I were given the address of the Infection Specialists Group. It was there that we would learn how to administer my Zosyn IV infusion at home. We were trained by a nurse who reviewed the steps and both my husband and I repeated the process to ensure we had it covered. The main emphasis was to make sure that the catheter was properly sterilized before use and to take the medication on time, which was every six hours. The prescription of the Zosyn antibiotic required IV administration every six hours using an elastomeric ball, which was refrigerated and had to be used within six hours of removal from the fridge. To make things easier, I created a flow chart for the Zosyn administration for us to follow.

April 2, 2019, Tuesday, 9:30 am

My Appendix Ruptured – I was not Told!

Due to my illness, I was now working while on bed rest. I remember this day like it was yesterday. It was Tuesday morning when the phone rang; it was the surgeon that my PCP had previously recommended. He was calling because I had missed my 9:00 am appointment

He was talking very fast and said, "Hi Dr. Johnson, this is Dr. Williams and I wanted to talk to you. I have reviewed your recent CT scan and I see that your appendix has ruptured and that you have a pool of phlegm in your abdomen. I just wanted to know when you would like to schedule your surgery."

I was once again in profound shock. "What do you mean that my appendix has ruptured?"

He glibly stated, "I have your second CT scan, it is clear that your appendix has ruptured."

I responded that I would need to call him back. I was numb and in complete disbelief. The thought of fecal matter from my colon traveling via my ruptured appendix into my abdomen was overwhelming. I immediately called my husband. I was very upset and felt my life coming apart and needed to collect myself as I explained the news that my appendix had ruptured. He recommended that I contact the Infection Specialist Group. I immediately contacted the office and asked to speak to the doctor, who was unavailable but I was able to speak to the physician assistant. I relayed my earlier conversation with the surgeon and I wanted to know if I needed to have surgery. He reiterated the need for my colon to heal, and that the IV antibiotic would help my body to heal. I ended the telephone call with much trepidation. I was deeply worried that I was not receiving the truth. I was resolved to continue to pray and maintain my faith in God.

April 9, 2019, Tuesday, 10:30 am

It was now Tuesday of the following week, the day that I had to pick up my Zosyn from the infection specialist's office. As I was leaving the office, I ran into the emergency room resident who was with the emergency room team during my second ER visit.

I confronted him. "Hi, do you have a minute?"

He responded, "Yes."

"I received a call from Dr. Williams from another hospital last week about my second CT scan who informed me that my appendix has ruptured and was the reason why my abdomen was filled with phlegmon, also known as "bacterial pus." Why didn't you inform me that my appendix ruptured when I was in the ER?"

He turned red and responded weakly, "We thought that it was best not to tell you."

He then quickly walked down the long corridor. I was infuriated and flabbergasted that the ER surgeons did not tell me the truth about my appendix. The CT scan clearly showed that there was bacterial pus in my abdomen from my ruptured appendix. This was blatant medical malpractice.

April 15, 2019, Monday, 9:00 am - Tax Day

The at-home Zosyn IV administration continued for two weeks. It was Tax Day, and I was feeling poorly. I had chills and a fever that was rising quickly. I was told that if I get a fever, it could be a PICC line infection, and I should immediately call the Infection Specialist Group. I urgently called the office and once again, I asked to speak to the doctor. Once again, he was not available. For the second time, I spoke to the physician assistant (PA) not the physician. "I am concerned that I have a fever, chills, and no appetite." The PA responded that I am scheduled for another CT scan and asked if I could visit the office that afternoon. I told him yes.

I arrived at the outpatient imaging center and learned that my CT scan order was faxed to the office. The technician was seemingly excited to administer the contrasting dye using my PICC line, but I failed to match her enthusiasm. I really wanted to know what was causing my fever to spike. After she completed the CT scan, and I got dressed to leave, she told me that the office will contact my doctor with the results. During the drive home I began a period of rumination followed by extreme consternation.

About two hours later, I received a call from the physician assistant, not the doctor. He informed me that I now have an abscess and I needed surgery immediately. He explained that the abscess will be removed by an interventional radiologist. I was trying to be astute and listen attentively, however, I was not prepared for a new ailment.

April 16, 2019, Tuesday, 9:00 am

The next morning, I had to go to the infection specialist's office to pick up a supply of the antibiotic, Zosyn. I woke up feeling lethargic but managed to drive myself to the office. I was met by the office administrative assistant, Kelly, a thin white woman, and asked her if the doctor was available to talk to him about my newly found abscess. The doctor was not available; however, I could speak to the physician's assistant. I also wanted to discuss my CT scan analysis that showed reduced inflammation in both my colon and appendix. Thus, to me, it was time for me to have my appendix removed. However, I had to wait to see the physician assistant

The next step of my office visit was to meet with the medical assistant to change the bandage for my PICC line. The medical assistant, Kendra, was a tall brown woman with a beautiful smile.

"How are you feeling?" she asked.

"Not well. I now have an abscess." I bemoaned.

She began taking my vitals; my blood pressure was elevated, and my temperature was 104 degrees-F, which was higher than the 101 degrees-F from yesterday. She was concerned. Kendra changed my bandage and escorted me to the physician assistant's office. As I sat in the sterile office with pale blue walls, I felt as though my body was shutting down. It was already four weeks since my first emergency room visit.

I was sitting on the bed with a copy of the spreadsheet with my three CT scans when the physician assistant arrived at the office.

"How are you feeling?" He asked.

"I do not feel well." I responded barely able to sit erect. He then proceeded to tell me that the Interventional Radiologist stated that he could not drain the abscess due to its location. I shared my CT scan spreadsheet that showed a reduction in inflammation in both my colon and appendix. He interrupted me and said, "You are very ill and need to get to the emergency room for surgery. You have a fever of 104 degrees-F. That appendix needs to come out today." I told him that I agree. I said a prayer of gratitude that my appendix would finally be removed.

CHAPTER 8: TAKING CONTROL – I NEED TO FIND A SURGEON

April 16, 2019, Tuesday, 10:30 am
My Third Emergency Room Visit

I called my husband, "Hi honey, I am at the infection specialist's office. My fever is now 104 degrees-F, and they are taking me to the emergency room. Please meet me there, okay."

"Okay, honey, I will see you there," he said.

I couldn't believe that this was my third visit to the emergency room! The office assistant took me by wheelchair to the emergency room, which is in an adjacent building. The buildings are connected by a long corridor. As I am being transported to the ER, my head was spinning as well as I felt miserable. My heart was pounding and I was sweating profusely. However, a part of me was also relieved. I have wanted that appendix out of my body for weeks and it will finally happen. Upon arrival at the ER, some of the nurses now recognized me and greeted me by name.

"Oh no, Dr. Johnson, you are back." I was officially a "frequent flyer." This is the name for patients who are in the emergency room at least once a week. I was taken to an examination room. My husband soon arrived and he could see that I was gravely ill. His concern for me was etched in his face as he said, "This is your third ER visit in four weeks. The appendectomy must be done today." I agreed emphatically.

Once again, I am examined by the same white male emergency room physician assistant, who also looked at me with great concern.

"You are very ill; you need that appendix removed today." He told me.

"Yes, my husband and I agree," I replied.

He then informed me that he had contacted the emergency surgery team and the surgery should occur very soon. I assumed that the operating room was being prepped for my surgery and I should be transported there in less than one hour.

The emergency room nurse started my IV and I was given pain medication. I anxiously waited to be taken to the operating room. Once again, an elderly white man entered my room and introduced himself as the ER Surgeon. He informed me that he just completed a consult with the infection specialist; the same specialist who had avoided my call for the past two weeks.

"We figured out the problem. We believe that you have developed an allergy to the antibiotic, Zosyn and have a Zosyn fever," he said.

"I spoke to the emergency room physician assistant and he stated that I would have an appendectomy. I am confused." The surgeon showed no empathy or compassion for my plight.

"I heard the nurse call you doctor. What kind of doctor are you?"

"My doctorate is in chemical engineering. When will I have the appendectomy, based on the CT scan that I had yesterday, my colon is no longer inflamed?" I asked.

He responded sarcastically, "Probably in the summer, June or July."

"So, I am supposed to keep the PICC line until June or July. I can't pick up my grandchildren, I can't exercise or work." The surgeon again, was stoic and didn't respond

By now, the infection specialist had arrived in my room.

I was not hopeful that the infection specialist would be able to convince the ER surgeon that I needed surgery as soon as possible. He introduced himself and advised me that he definitely believed that I was having an allergic reaction to the Zosyn.

"Why am I allergic? How many patients have allergic reactions to Zosyn?"

"What antibiotic will replace the Zosyn, and what is the probability that it will fail?" I asked him.

At that moment he said that they will try Rocephin because it can be administered at home like Zosyn.

"Why can't I just have the surgery?" I further inquired.

He responded, "I think that the Rocephin will work."

My husband and I were both stunned. We were baffled why the surgery was being postponed for the third time! This was the third surgeon that had refused to perform my appendectomy.

The next steps were for me to be admitted to the hospital and get started on the new antibiotic. Once my fever was addressed, I was allowed to go home with the PICC line.

We finally arrived at the unit around 10:00 pm. By that time my husband and I are both utterly tired and exasperated. This time we were taken to a different surgical unit. I had worked with the nurse manager on the Acute Appendicitis Surgical Care Plan. I informed my husband that I had a plan to ensure that I get my appendectomy and not wait for two to three months.

"I will meet with the nurse manager first thing in the morning and schedule a consult with the same colorectal surgeon who did my husband's colon cancer surgery."

He replied, "Great plan, honey."

April 17, 2019, Wednesday, 7:00 am

The next morning, I was ready to execute my plan. I wanted to have a consult with the colorectal surgeon and get this appendix out of me. While, waiting to meet with the nurse manager, my friend, Kay called me. She is a nurse and had been following me for the past few weeks. "I am just calling to check on you to see if you had the surgery yesterday." She was concerned that I was developing sepsis since my appendix had already ruptured and the Zosyn did not work. At that moment I became thoroughly afraid for my life. For the most part, bacterial infections are most often to blame for sepsis. But what I find most compelling, is that it can also happen because of other infections. It can begin anywhere bacteria, parasites, fungi, or viruses can enter or develop in your body.,

In the hospital, my experience reminded me that when hospitalized, bacteria may enter through IV lines, surgical wounds, urinary catheters, and bed sores. Sepsis is more common in people who:

- Have weakened immune systems because of conditions like HIV or cancer or because they take drugs such as steroids or those that prevent rejection of transplanted organs

- Are pregnant
- Are very young
- Are elderly, especially if they have other health problems
- Were recently hospitalized or had major surgeries
- Use catheters or breathing tubes
- Have diabetes
- Have a serious medical condition such as appendicitis, pneumonia, meningitis, cirrhosis, or a urinary tract infection

I was very worried that I had sepsis. I would later learn, after reading my medical records thoroughly, that I did have sepsis and I also had internal bleeding. In retrospect, it was by the grace of God that I was alive and able to take action.

Meeting with the Nurse Manager and Colorectal Surgeon

I truly did not sleep well due to the constant interruptions by the nursing staff. I was still very ill. I had not been able to eat normally for weeks, and I had lost ten pounds. I got out of my hospital bed and walked to the nurse manager's office with my IV pole in tow. I knew her over the past five years, as we had worked on multiple projects together.

It was now 7:30 am and the nurse manager looked at me with grave concern. She then stated, "I have reviewed your case and I can't believe that you did not have the appendectomy. You should have had surgery by now. Do you want a consult, or do you want to have the colorectal surgeon take over your case?" I paused because initially, I was thinking of a consult, but to have a new surgeon assigned to my case and replace the arrogant emergency room surgeon was the better option. I stated, "Yes, I prefer that the colorectal surgeon take over my case."

I call my husband with the good news that I will meet with his surgeon. Later in the day, the colorectal surgeon came to my room and I reminded him that he did my husband's cancer surgery thirteen years ago. He stated, "I reviewed your case, what do you want me to do?" It told him that I want him to perform the appendectomy. "Yes, I can do that. I will schedule your surgery." I thanked him and felt relieved that, after a month of severe illness, I was finally getting the surgery that my body needed. In my mind, I thought that I would have surgery the next day.

April 18, 2019, Thursday
Not so Fast – My Surgery was Delayed

The next day, I was anxiously awaiting the surgery to be scheduled. However, that was not to happen. The morning rounds began, and the surgical resident assigned to my case provided me with a new plan. The sad news was that I could not have surgery because my white blood cell count was too low and needed to be increased. I explained to the surgeon that like millions of Black Americans, historically, I have a low white blood cell count and was healthy until the acute appendicitis. I was being treated like a cancer patient on chemotherapy.

Because I had my laptop, I printed my lab reports for the past five years. Ironically, my white blood cell count was actually higher at 3.4 than my 2017 lab results which was 2.4. To no avail, my surgery was delayed, and the surgeon ordered Neupogen, a medication usually given to chemotherapy patients, to help me increase my white blood cell count.

Later that day, a new infection specialist came to my room for a consult.

He stated, "I hear that you are "angry" that your surgery has been delayed."

So, I was the "angry Black woman" who was being unreasonable. The racist "angry black woman" trope has been used throughout history to discount and diminish our outrage at racist behavior. I was too tired to argue and simply responded that I was healthy with a low white blood cell count. I was surprised when he agreed.

He mentioned a research study that was authored years ago that made the argument that Black Americans should not be judged by white healthcare guidelines. He went on to say that the health metrics created 50 years ago were based on data from college-aged white men and needed to be updated. He also referred to the low white blood cell count as "benign ethnic neutropenia." Of course, the researcher in me had to look up this term. The response by the Black medical community was outraged that white racist health metrics were used to define what was normal for Black people as a disease. There were also studies that proved how Black women with low white blood cell counts were denied chemotherapy for breast cancer when needed. This delay in care resulted in a delay in treatment and thereby poor health outcomes.[79] The next day, my white blood cell count increased to 3.8 which is in the normal range and my surgery is scheduled for the upcoming Friday, April 19, 2019.

Surgery – At Last!
April 19, 2019, Friday at 6:00 am

The day for my surgery had finally arrived. I could not believe it was nearly five weeks since my first emergency room visit. The surgeon explained to us that the plan was to perform the surgery laparoscopically by creating three small holes in my abdomen. The surgery should take approximately one hour. I was transported to the operating room (OR) for the surgery.

The next thing that I remember was my husband trying to wake me up and I was shivering. "Is it over?" I asked. "Yes," he responded. We were in the post-anesthesia recovery unit and remained there until I was cleared for transport back to my hospital room. Later that day, one of the surgeons came to my room. He was a middle-aged East Indian man who I did not know. He looked at me with worried eyes. He revealed that my surgery was very complicated because my appendix was no longer attached to my colon. In fact, my ruptured appendix was necrotic and actually in multiple pieces throughout my belly. In order for the surgeons to get all the pieces, an incision down my belly was needed. Once my belly was opened, every organ was covered with bacteria. Once they removed every piece of my appendix, they had to wash my belly with an antibiotic-containing solution multiple times to remove the tremendous number of bacteria. He then said, "You are very lucky to be alive." I told him that I agree wholeheartedly, and I then asked him, "What is my prognosis?" He declared that I have a long road ahead. The main goal was to make sure that the bacteria was addressed. Due to the huge number of bacteria in my body, I needed to remain on an antibiotic for two weeks and remain in the hospital for a week to receive the antibiotics intravenously, after which I should be able to go home on oral medication.

I was not surprised by his assessment that I was "lucky to be alive." I also knew that I was gravely ill and needed surgery. Had I not listened to my inner voice that told me to use my "voice" and find the right surgeon, I would be dead. This was a life-changing event; being that close to death and knowing that my nightmare could have been easily prevented.

The road to recovery was not easy and it took a year for my body to fully heal. My primary care physician told me to sue for medical malpractice and that she would be my witness. I prayed about that action and decided to file a complaint with the hospital patient and family experience department. The complaint was in the form of a simple phone call to the department's director, a white woman who I did not know. She listened attentively as I shared with her my three emergency room visits and how I almost died due to multiple delays of my appendectomy. She informed me that an investigation would be performed followed by a debrief with me. I was not involved in the investigation.

The debrief was held four months after my surgery in a small dimly lit conference room. All of the faces were white. There was an elderly white male surgeon, a middle-aged white emergency room physician, and the white Patient Relations Department director. I knew the white surgeon and ER physician from previous projects that I worked on as a healthcare consultant. The surgeon began with an apology for my experience. I came prepared. I had all of my data summarized, along with all of the physician notes that I downloaded from the patient portal. I had reviewed the physician's notes and they were filled with lies. In some cases, addendums were added months later to update the narratives. It was the institution's response to a pending lawsuit.

I began the debrief with my overview of my healthcare nightmare.

I stated, "I was the project leader for the Acute Appendicitis Surgical Care Plan that requires the patient to be transported to the Operating Room within 8 hours after the CT scan that confirms an acute appendicitis. Why was my surgery delayed?" The response by the surgeon was that "conservative management" can be used to allow the appendix to calm down.

I then asked, "Do you agree that the gold standard for acute appendicitis is the surgical removal of the appendix?"

The surgeon did not respond to my question, but instead deflected to the successful cases of conservative management.

I responded, "My sister-in-law was diagnosed with acute appendicitis and sent home with antibiotics and died of a ruptured appendix. I went to the Emergency Room three times and was denied a surgical intervention by the ER surgeons. How many Black patients, have had successful outcomes with conservation management?"

The emergency room physician responded that he did not know but will get the data.

Throughout the debrief, they apologized for my experience, but they did not take accountability for their actions. The meeting ended with their assurance that they will review the conservative management data.

I was dissatisfied and told the director that I wanted the data. I later found out that there was no way to collect the data because they generally do not track which patient receives conservative management.

This is the challenge with healthcare data. It is structured for billing the patient for services and not for research and analysis. I really needed the data to demonstrate racial bias regarding my treatment.

My husband and I weighed the pros and cons of filing a medical malpractice lawsuit. The pros are that we will hold the hospital accountable for my near-death experience. The primary con was that I was a healthcare consultant working at the same hospital where the malpractice occurred. I told my husband that we should pray on it. After long prayer and contemplation, I am grateful to be alive and decided not to pursue legal action. It is a decision that I deeply regret. Why? It is imperative that Black people find their voices and take action when they receive poor healthcare. As such, I have created the Patient's Advocate Toolkit to help Black families navigate the American healthcare system.

PART 3

PATIENT ADVOCATE TOOLKIT FOR YOUR SURVIVAL

VOICE YOUR CONCERNS™ FOR YOUR HEALTHCARE TOOLKIT

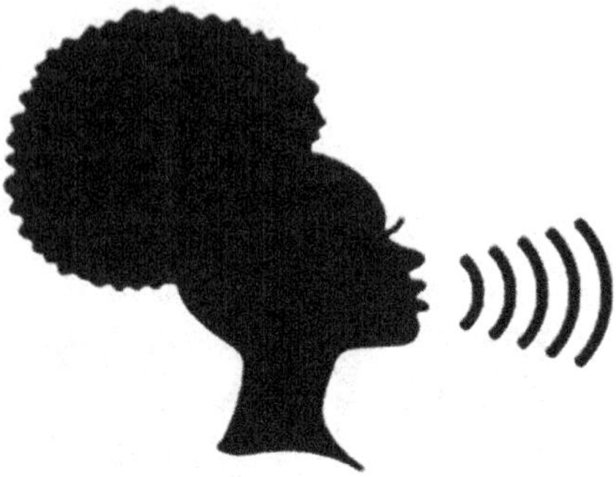

This toolkit was created for Black women who are patients, caregivers, or patient advocates and have concerns about both healthcare and how they are being treated. Read on to learn about how healthcare delivery works, your rights as a patient, and who to contact if you are not getting the quality healthcare that you and your family deserve.

What is the Voice Your Concerns™ about Your Healthcare Toolkit?

As a healthcare consultant working at hospitals and physician office practices for over ten years, I was responsible for analyzing problems and identifying solutions for myriad healthcare problems. I worked with various project teams that included physicians, nurses, patient care technicians, administrations, office staff, and patients and used a "Voice of the Customer" model to ensure that all solutions would be sustained. As a patient, I nearly died after being sent home with acute appendicitis and antibiotics instead of having life-saving surgery. The doctors did not value me as a Black woman and informed me that my excruciating pain was not that bad. Upon surviving my horrific ordeal, God told me to create this toolkit to help Black women understand how to become patient advocates. I pray that you will use the tools and information to help you navigate the complex healthcare system.

If you are experiencing healthcare challenges including delays in care or you feel that you are not receiving the care you deserve, this toolkit is for you. If you need assistance on how to use this toolkit or like to share your feedback, I would love to hear from you at: Voiceyourconcerns12@gmail.com.

Table of Contents

Patient Bill of Rights

I would guess that you are not aware that you have basic rights, protected by Federal and State laws when you need access to healthcare. In 1973, the American Hospital Association (AHA) created the Patient Bill of Rights.[80] In March 2010, under President Barack Obama, the Patient Protection and Affordable Care Act, known as "ACA" or "Obamacare" provided more healthcare protections including:[81]

1. Insurance plans must cover people with pre-existing conditions.
2. Insurance plans must provide free preventive care including annual check-ups and screenings.
3. Young adults can remain on parents' insurance plan until age 26.
4. Ends lifetime and yearly dollars limits on insurance coverage.
5. Protects your choice of doctor.

Your patient rights are protected by federal and state law as summarized below. Each time you go to the emergency room, hospital, or physician's office, please use your phone to review their Patient Bill of Rights. Although they may be slightly tweaked, all should include the following rights.

The Patient Bill of Rights is summarized below: [80]

1. Receive care that is respectful of your personal beliefs, culture and spiritual values.
2. An explanation in terms that you can understand and have any question answered concerning your symptoms, diagnosis, prognosis, and treatment.
3. Appropriate assessment and management of your symptoms, including pain.

4. Know your diagnosis; prognosis; testing and treatment to be used; risks of treatment and common side effects of medications; financial considerations associated with medical care
5. Know the contents of your medical records through interpretation by the provider.
6. Know your healthcare team.
7. Develop a collaborative plan to prevent your medical problem from recurring.
8. Choose or change your provider.
9. Refuse to be examined or treated and to be informed of the consequence of such decisions.
10. Be assured of the confidential treatment of disclosures and records and to approve or refuse the release of such information, except when the release of specific information is required by law or is necessary to safeguard you or the university community.
11. Be informed and provide consent to participate in research.
12. Participate in the consideration of ethical issues that may arise in the provision of your care.
13. Provide feedback on the services you receive and not be penalized for that feedback.
14. Have access to the Patient Portal to review your medical records that include all healthcare encounters. You can also request your medical records from your healthcare provider, and they should be provided to you within 30 days.

15.

Who is Who in Healthcare? – Roles and Responsibilities

It is important to understand who provides your care during your healthcare encounter. The tables below list the roles and responsibilities of both emergency room (also known as the emergency department (ED)) staff and the hospital.

Tips for your Emergency Room visit regarding Roles and Responsibilities
When you go to the emergency room or emergency department, it is important for you to understand the healthcare roles and responsibilities. A healthcare emergency is a challenging time for you as a patient or family member. Remember to take notes during the visit and record the names of each person involved in your care delivery.

Tips for your Hospital visit regarding Roles and Responsibilities
After an emergency room visit or traumatic event, you may have to be hospitalized. It is important to understand the different roles that are responsible for your healthcare during your visit. Please be aware that the hospital staff works 8-hour or 12-hour shifts. The nurse that you have in the morning will not be the same nurse in the evening. The tests that you may need may not be available during the evening and you may have to wait until the next day to get that test. Also, during the weekend, there may be reduced staff thus,

the tests that were ordered on Friday, may not be performed until Monday. As always, take notes during your hospital stay and record the names of each person involved in your care. In your hospital room, there should be a whiteboard that lists the names of staff during that shift. You can use your cell phone and take a picture of the whiteboard during each shift to know who provided your care.

Table 1.

Emergency Room (ER)/Emergency Department (ED) Roles & Responsibilities

Role	Responsibilities
Triage Nurse	A triage nurse is generally the first medical professional that a patient sees when they are taken into an emergency room, according to the Center for Advancing Health. It will be the triage nurse's job to assess whether or not the patient needs immediate care or can wait. The triage nurse is the gatekeeper. The triage nurse will also enter your complaint into the system.
ER Nurse	An ED nurse is generally the next medical professional that the patient will see in the emergency room. The ED Nurse will be responsible for taking care of the patient during the ER visit.
Billing Coordinator	Responsible for obtaining your insurance information and who will be responsible for the ER visit bill. The data is entered into the EMR (Electronic Management Record).
ER Physician	Responsible for examining the patient and ordering the necessary tests to determine your diagnosis and treatment.

Role	Responsibilities
ER Physician Assistant	The ER physician assistant is a clinician who may also perform the examination and order lab work and tests that will be used to determine your diagnosis and treatment.
ER Surgeon	Responsible for performing emergency surgery for either a trauma-related admission or after a consult order by the emergency room physician.
ER Radiologist	Responsible for reviewing and interpreting your imaging tests including: X-rays, CT scans, MRIs, and Ultrasounds.
ER Patient Care Technician	Responsible for assisting the ER nurse and staff with the patient including taking vitals and caring for the patient. The PCT will perform administrative tasks if needed.
Social Worker	Responsible for working with the patient to identify what is needed for a safe discharge to home, nursing facility, or hospital. Can also identify community resources that are needed to support the patient and family.
Case Manager	A nurse that is responsible for reviewing the case needs of the patient and family including insurance coverage for home health services, facilities, medical equipment, i.e., oxygen tank, walker, wheelchair, etc.
Behavioral Health Specialist	Responsible for assisting patients that are having a behavioral health crisis and ensuring that behavioral health needs are met. Don't hesitate to ask for a behavioral health specialist if needed.
ED Patient Escort	Responsible for transporting the patient to stations throughout the hospital system including imaging, laboratory, infusion, inpatient Room, etc.
Behavioral Health Nurse	Responsible for performing a mental health assessment to keep both patient and staff safe. The BH nurse will coordinate the placement in a mental health facility if needed.

Table 2.

Hospital Roles & Responsibilities

Role	Responsibilities
Patient Escort	Responsible for transporting the patient to stations throughout the hospital system including Imaging, Laboratory, Infusion, Inpatient Room, etc. The transport can be done via wheelchair or stretcher.
House-keeper	Responsible for cleaning and sanitizing your hospital room daily. Room cleanliness is critical so that you do not get an HAI (Hospital Acquired Infection) during your visit. Infections include COVID-19, C-Diff, MRSA, etc.
Patient Care Technician	Responsible for providing your care including measuring your vitals, helping you get out of bed, and walk with you to the bathroom, and help with your daily hygiene.
Bedside Nurse	Responsible for the care transition from the emergency room (ER) to your inpatient visit. The bedside nurse will complete a communication (called a Handoff) with the ER nurse and hospital nurse during your visit. The handoff during a shift change should be completed in your presence if you are able. This will make sure that the shared information is accurate. The bedside nurse may have a total of 5 to 7 patients depending on the hospital. A Critical Care Bedside Nurse will only have 1 to 2 patients. The bedside nurse is also responsible for your care, administering your medication, and communicating your request to meet with physicians and specialists.

Role	Responsibilities
Charge Nurse	Responsible for managing the activities of the unit (ward) staff during the shift. A shift maybe 8 to 12 hours. This is the person to contact if you have a complaint about your care and the nurse manager is not available.
Nurse Manager	Responsible for leading the unit staff and ensuring that all care is delivered in a safe and caring manner. This is the person to contact if you have a complaint or a question regarding your care.
Hospitalist / Nurse Practitioner	Responsible for your care and discharge during your hospital visit. They will create your Plan of Care (POC), and order medications and tests. If the hospital does not have this role, your primary care physician, surgeon or specialist will be responsible for care and discharge. They will examine you daily and record your progress in the Electronic Management Record (EMR).
Specialists	Physicians who are consulted on your case and may include, a cardiologist, a pulmonologist, an oncologist, etc. A consult will be ordered by the hospitalist.
Patient & Family Services Director	Responsible for managing all complaints from either the patient or family regarding care delivery.
Therapists	The hospitalist may order treatment from a respiratory therapist, physical therapist, or speech therapist depending on your illness.
Case Manager	A nurse that is responsible for reviewing the case needs of the patient and family including insurance coverage for home health

Role	Responsibilities
	services, facilities, medical equipment, i.e., oxygen tank, walker, wheelchair, etc.
Social Worker	Responsible for working with the patient to identify what is needed for a safe discharge to home, nursing facility, or hospital. Can also identify community resources that are needed to support the patient and family.
Dietary Assistant	Responsible for taking your food order for breakfast, lunch, and dinner.

Healthcare Workflows

Once you understand the roles and responsibilities of the healthcare staff, the next item to understand is how your healthcare is delivered. For over a decade, I have created myriad healthcare workflows also known as process maps. What I do that is unique, is that I show who is responsible for the activity during the process. Please review the workflows and think about your role as the patient and what you can do to make sure that you receive the best quality care possible. The three important workflows include:

Doctor Appointment Workflow

When you go to your doctor's appointment whether it is a primary care physician, or a specialist for example a cardiologist, nephrologist, oncologist, gynecologist, obstetrician, etc., it is important to understand who does what during your visit by reviewing the workflow in Figure 1.

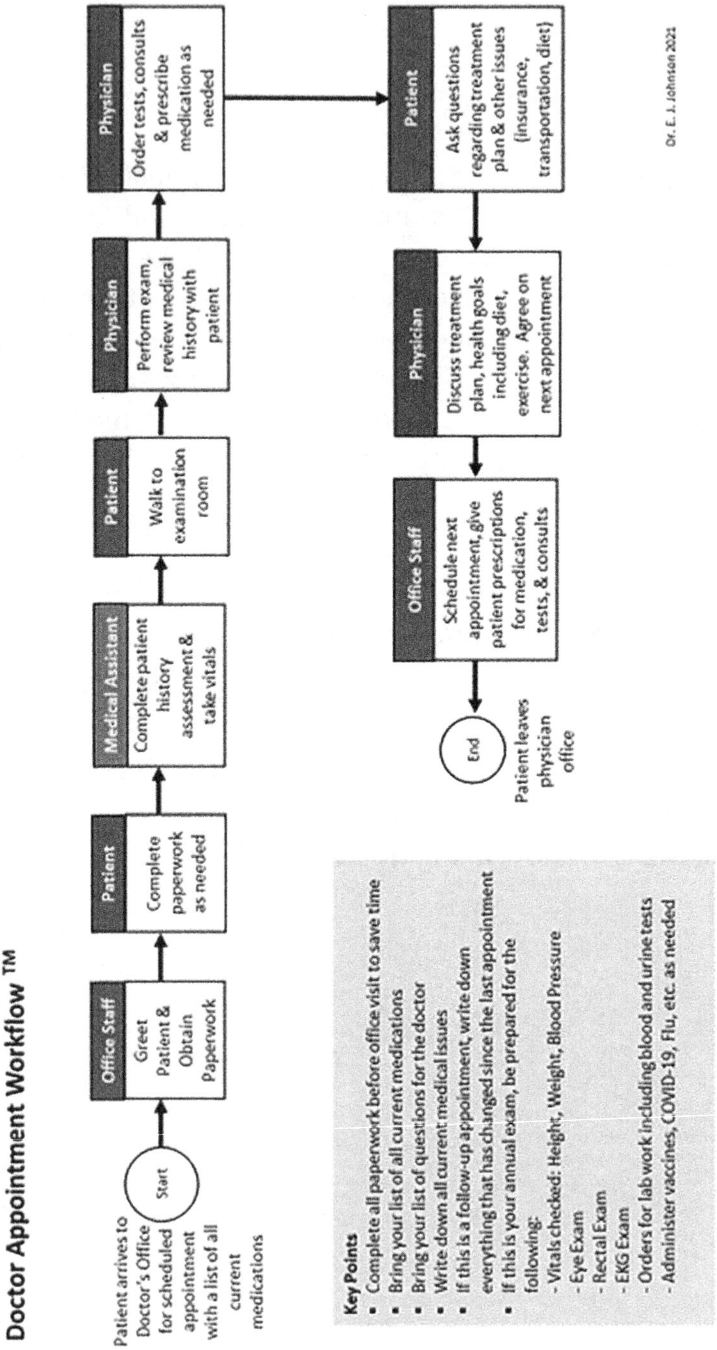

Figure 1. Doctor Appointment Workflow

Key Points

1. Either complete all paperwork before the office visit or arrive early to the appointment to do so to save time, if not your visit may not begin on time.

2. Bring your list of all current medications to let the doctor know what medications you are on and how often you take them.

3. Bring your list of questions for the doctor to make sure that they are discussed during your appointment.

4. Write down all current medical issues to include in your conversations.

5. If this is a follow-up appointment, write down everything that has changed since the last appointment to make sure that the doctor is aware.

Emergency Room /Department Workflow

When you go to the emergency room, it is important to understand who does what during your visit by reviewing the workflow in Figure 2.

Key Points

1. The Emergency Severity Index (ESI) determines the patient's level of care on a scale from 1 to 5 with 1 meaning that the patient needs immediate medical intervention due to a life-threatening situation and a 5 meaning that the patient has a non-urgent medical emergency. If you

feel that your medical needs are not being met, ask to speak to the emergency room nurse manager.

2. Research data shows that ER staff's racial bias can impact the level of care for Black patients. This is a huge problem as demonstrated by data about COVID-19 patients. Please use your voice and speak up about how you are being treated immediately.

3. Research data shows that a Black patient's pain levels may be dismissed due to centuries of racism and dehumanization.

4. Research data shows that Black patients can leave the emergency room without treatment due to longer wait times.

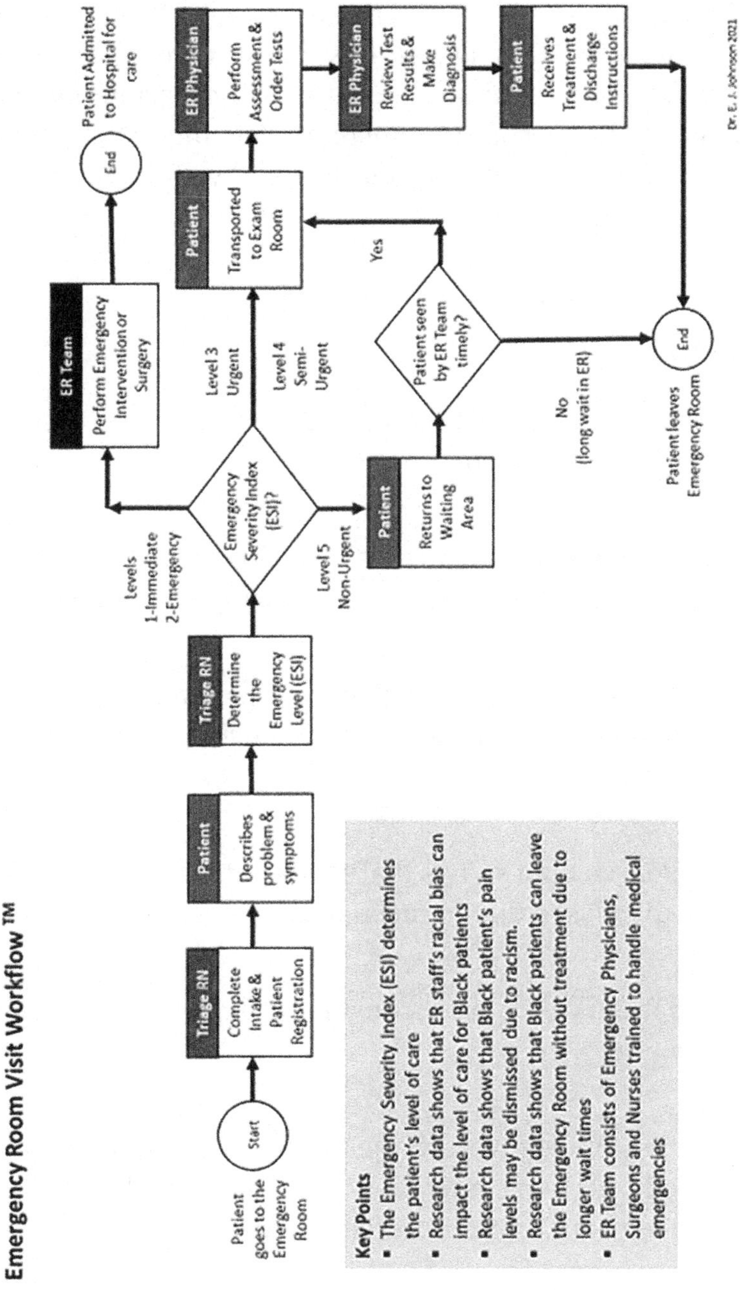

Figure 2. Emergency Room Visit Workflow

Hospital Admission and Discharge Workflow

Once you go to the emergency room, you may have to be admitted to the hospital. During your hospital stay, your care team will develop your care plan and a doctor will determine when you can be discharged from the hospital. It is important to understand who does what during your hospital visit by reviewing the workflow in Figure 3.

Key Points

1. Bedside Nurse is responsible for administering care including medication.

2. Research data shows that racial bias can impact the level of care Black patients receive during hospital visits.

3. Research data shows that Black patients' requests for consults with physicians and specialists can be ignored by staff.

4. Research data shows that Black patients' pain levels may be dismissed due to racial bias.

5. A patient can request consults with physicians and family members.

6. Patient meets with Home Health Nurse to review health needs at home and any equipment including walker, wheelchair, oxygen, crutches, etc.

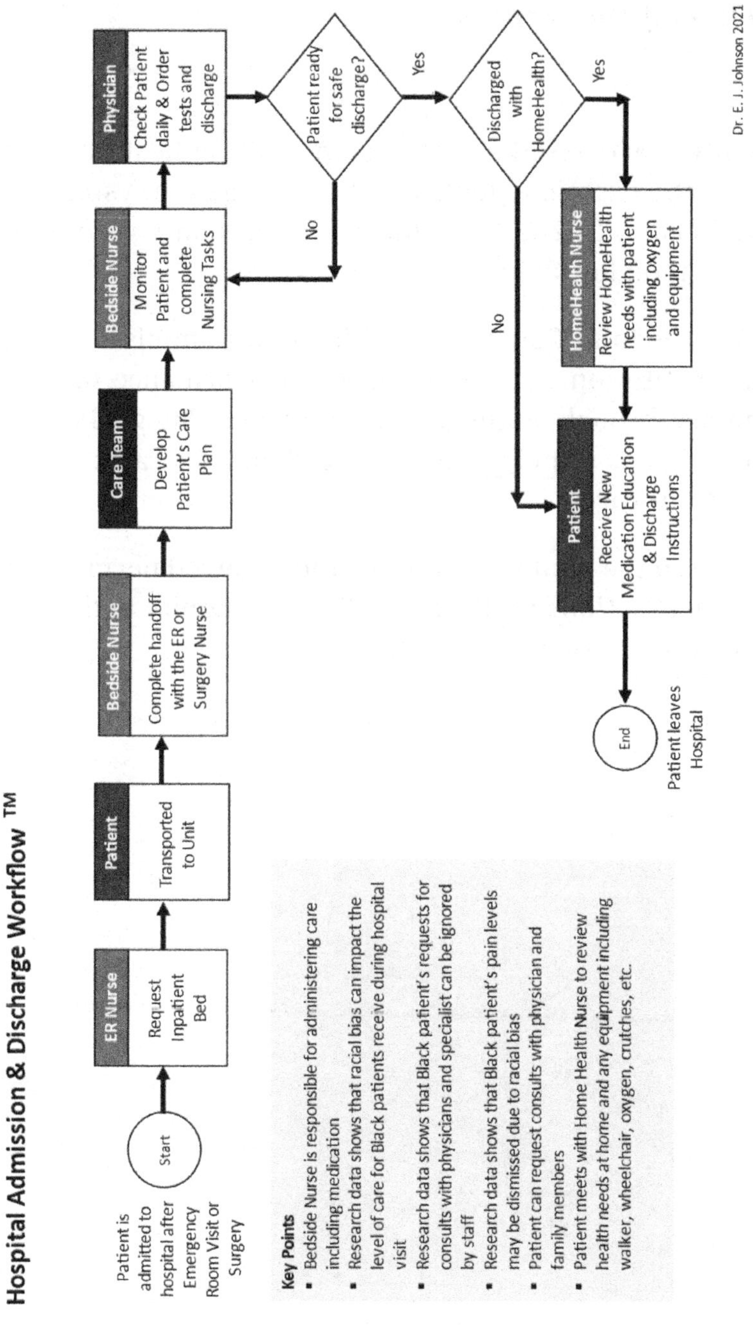

Figure 3. Hospital Admission and Discharge Workflow

The Fight for Racial Justice and Equity – Black Patients and Racial Disparities

Recently, I witnessed an astonishing shift in healthcare leaders who for the first time publicly acknowledge the systemic racism in healthcare. In 2021, the Joint Commission issued an official statement on Racial Justice and Equity. [82]

What is the Joint Commission? The Joint Commission is the national institution that monitors the performance of American Hospitals through audits and certification. The goal of the Joint Commission is to help patients and their advocates become active in their care.

I contacted the Joint Commission and received permission to include their actions on Racial Justice and Equity and how to report discrimination as noted below.

The Joint Commission Stands for Racial Justice and Equity
– Printed with Permission

The Joint Commission has been deeply shaken and saddened by the death of George Floyd. The image of his senseless death is a cause for all of us to examine our institutions to assure we are working toward eliminating racial inequality, bias, and disparities in America.

The Joint Commission has no tolerance for racial discrimination in our organization or in the health care organizations we accredit and certify.

Sadly, we know that racism exists in health care. Many decades ago, Dr. Martin Luther King Jr. said, "Of all the forms of inequality, injustice in health care is the most shocking and inhumane." Yet, we continue to see racial bias and disparities in care received by people of color.

People of color in America often experience significantly poorer health outcomes than their white counterparts. Black mothers are nearly four times more likely to die during pregnancy, during childbirth, and immediately following their pregnancies than white mothers.

While data is still incomplete regarding the coronavirus, we can see that African Americans are dying at twice the expected rate based on their share of the population nationwide. In some states, they are dying at three to four times the expected rate. And given the low access to testing in Black communities, these numbers may be higher.

Institutional, systemic racism adversely affects health. Studies have shown that racism and its associated stressors begin impacting physical and mental health as early as childhood and adolescence, leading to poor mental health and higher rates of chronic disease later in life.

The Joint Commission is committed to safe, high-quality health care for all. We require our accredited organizations to protect the rights of individuals and prohibit discrimination. Our patient-centered communication standards guide providers to assure that people of all races, backgrounds, disabilities, and income levels receive care that is free of prejudice.

But none of us acting alone can solve this problem. This is a challenge that dates to our country's founding. The only way to overcome it will be to work together.

We ask all health care workers, patients, and families to speak up if they see an injustice committed. Health care organizations should encourage and support their staff to confront overt racism and implement efforts to address the implicit biases of coworkers and senior staff members.

If you experience discrimination at an accredited organization, tell us. You can submit a report of what happened to our Office of Quality and Patient Safety online, here.

Clinicians take an oath to do no harm. We think it is time for all of us to take one, too — to cast away prejudice and stand with all people of color in ending racism and injustice.

Now, let's work together to put an end to this plague.

https://www.jointcommission.org/resources/news-and-multimedia/the-joint-commission-stands-for-racial-justice-and-equity/

How to Report Healthcare Discrimination to the Joint Commission
– Printed with Permission

It is undeniable that racism can harm patients' health. This directly opposes the Joint Commission's mission and vision to help accredited and certified organizations provide safe, high-quality health care for all people. The Joint Commission has standards to guide its organizations and help ensure that all people receive care that is free from discrimination. The Joint Commission has no tolerance for bias or discrimination in its organizations. But we also know that institutional, systemic racism and bias still exist in health care. Differences in the quality of care received by patients or barriers and impediments to care can be due to:

- Race or ethnicity
- Age
- Gender identity or expression
- Geographic location
- Language
- Physical or mental ability
- Education level
- Religion or culture
- Sexual orientation
- Social and/or economic status
- Access to care or lack of resources, such as Internet or transportation

What to do

If you feel you are being discriminated against and are experiencing substandard care, speak up! You can do so by:

- Finding out about the hospital or health care organization's policy for reporting complaints. If possible, try to work with the organization.

- ➢ Talking to the organization's patient advocacy department (sometimes also called the patient liaison office or the patient advocacy team).

- ➢ Filing a complaint with the Office for Civil Rights, which is part of the U.S. Department of Health and Human Services, or with your state's health department.

    - ✓ Learn more about filing a complaint at: https://www.hhs.gov/civil-rights/filing-a-complaint/index.html.
    - ✓ File a complaint at: https://ocrportal.hhs.gov/ocr/smartscreen/main.jsf.

- ➢ Contacting the U.S. Department of Justice's Civil Rights Division.
    - ✓ By phone: 202-514-3847
    - ✓ By phone device for the deaf (TTY): 202-514-0716

If your issue remains unaddressed and the organization is accredited or certified by The Joint Commission, you can speak up by reporting the patient safety concern to us

- ✓ Online at: https://apps.jointcommission.org/QMSInternet/IncidentEntry.aspx

- ✓ By mail: Office of Quality and Patient Safety
  The Joint Commission One Renaissance Boulevard
  Oakbrook Terrace, Illinois 60181

Everyone deserves to be treated with respect. If you feel you are experiencing racist or discriminatory actions, speak up. By doing so, you may be helping future patients.

New Speak Up™ Against Discrimination campaign from The Joint Commission 10/05/2021. The Joint Commission today released Speak Up™ Against Discrimination, a new educational campaign that encourages patients to speak up if discriminated against while receiving health care. The campaign comes at a time when the COVID-19 pandemic has brought health inequities and disparities to the forefront

https://www.jointcommission.org/search/#q=racism&t=_Tab_All&sort=relevancy&f:_SitesOrganizations=[The%20Joint%20Commission]

About Your Health and Safety

It can be challenging for some Black women to find their voices during healthcare visits. You may be easily intimidated by authority figures including doctors and administrators. If your gut tells you something is not right, listen to your inner voice. Do not be afraid to voice your concerns to physicians, nurses, or office staff who demean, devalue or disrespect you. Do not worry if there will be repercussions against you because oftentimes you must fight to save lives. The death from the global pandemic corona virus, COVID-19, can occur quickly upon an emergency room visit. It may take only days or even hours for death to occur, thus you must find your voice and take prompt action.

Research shows that patients who take part in decisions about their healthcare are more likely to have better outcomes. However, for Black patients, the healthcare encounter may involve healthcare providers who may be or may not be aware of their racial biases. It is important that you ask questions about clinical decisions that impact your health. It is also critical that you ask questions to find out if there are resources and programs for your illness that are typically not shared with Black patients.

I have defined the VOICE Acronym as follows:

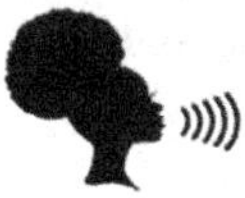

Voice Your Concerns and Don't Be Afraid to Speak Up

- Your health is very important. Voice your concerns and don't worry about being embarrassed if you don't understand something that your doctor, nurse, or other healthcare professional tells you.
- Your safety is important. Voice your concerns about safety. If you're having surgery, ask the doctor to mark the area that is to be operated on.
- Tell the nurse or the doctor if you think you are about to get the wrong medication.
- Tell the healthcare professionals if you think they have confused you with another patient.
- Contact the hospital patient relations department if you feel that your concerns are not addressed.

Own the Moment

Own the Moment and be Aware of What is Happening and the Actions that Impact your Safety

- During every healthcare encounter, make sure that you Own the Moment by being aware of what is going on. Pay attention to everything that is happening.
- Make sure that you know the names of each healthcare worker. Look at their badges (ID) and record their names. If you do not know the person, ask for their ID.
- Check to make sure that you are getting the correct treatment and the correct medication ordered by a licensed medical professional. Do not make assumptions.

- Make sure that the healthcare worker washes their hands. Hand washing is the most important way to prevent infections including COVID-19. Don't be afraid to ask the doctor or nurse to wash their hands in front of you. If you are in the hospital, please make sure that your visitors wash their hands in front of you.
- If you are in the hospital, know the time of day for your medications and make sure that you get them on time. Please tell the doctor or nurse if you did not get your medication.
- Take notes of the medical decisions regarding your care including new medications.
- Ask the nurse to review all medications with you and tell you about all possible side effects.
- Whenever you get a new medication, tell your doctors and nurses about allergies you have, or negative reactions you have had to other medicines.
- Ask about why you should take the medicine. Ask for written information about it, including its brand and generic names. Also, ask about the side effects of all medicines.
- If you do not recognize a medicine, double-check that it is for you. Ask about medicines that you are to take by mouth before you swallow them. Read the contents of the bags of intravenous (IV)fluids. If you're not well enough to do this, ask your advocate to do it.
- If you are given an IV, ask the nurse how long it should take for the liquid to run out. Tell the nurse if it doesn't seem to be dripping right (too fast or too slow).
- If you are taking a lot of medicines, be sure to ask your doctor or pharmacist if it is safe to take those medicines together. Do the same for vitamins, herbs, and over-the-counter medicines.

- Carry an up-to-date list of the medicines you are taking in your wallet or purse. Write down how much you take and when you take each medicine. Review your medicine list with your healthcare providers.

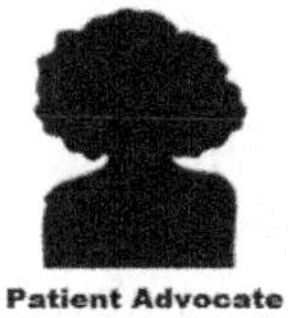

Include a Trusted Family Member or Friend to Serve as your Patient Advocate

- When you are under stress you may not be able to ask important healthcare questions. Your advocate can ask questions on your behalf.
- When you are in the hospital, find out if your patient advocate can stay with you during all consults with doctors, and even overnight. You will be able to rest better when someone you trust is there with you.
- Your advocate can help make sure you get the right medicines and treatments.
- Your advocate can also help remember answers to questions you have asked.
- Your advocate can write down the information you need to remember to voice your concerns when you cannot speak for yourself.
- Make sure this person understands what you expect from the healthcare encounter. Make sure your advocate knows your "Advance Directive" includes what you want to be done about life support and other lifesaving efforts if you are unconscious and not likely to get better.
- Your advocate should be someone who is not intimidated and can communicate well with healthcare professionals. This will help you get the best care.
- Your advocate should know your healthcare proxy decision-maker if you are assigned one. For example, you

may assign a family member to be your proxy. A proxy is a person you choose to sign a legal document to enable that person to make decisions about your healthcare when you are not able to make your own decisions. Your advocate may be your proxy. This person should know this ahead of time.

- Go over the consents for treatment including surgery with your advocate before you sign them. Make sure you both understand the treatment plan. If you do not, ask questions before you sign the consent form.
- Make sure your advocate understands the type of care you will need when you get home. If you do not have support at home, make sure that you get home healthcare service at home from a visiting nurse. Your advocate should know what to look for if your condition is getting worse. This person should also know whom to call for help.

Communicate with all Healthcare Providers about your Care Plan and your Illness

- You and your doctor should agree on exactly what will be done during each step of your care. If you want your advocate to be present, ask them to call your patient advocate/family member to listen to the care plan over the phone.
- Know who will be taking care of you. Know how long the treatment will last. Know how you should feel once you begin treatment.
- Understand that more tests or medicines may not always be better for you. Ask your doctor how a new test or medicine will help or hinder your health or quality of life.

- Keep copies of your medical records from your other hospital stays and share them with your healthcare team. This will give them better information about your health history.
- Don't be afraid to seek a second opinion about your health. If you are unsure about the best treatment for your illness, feel free to talk with one or two additional doctors. The more information that you have about all kinds of treatment available to you, the better you will feel about the decision made.
- Ask your doctor what resources are available for your illness including a nurse navigator, clinical trial, support groups, and home health services. A support group may help you prepare for your patient journey. The group members may be able to tell you what to expect and what worked best for them.
- Talk to your doctor and family about your wishes for resuscitation and other life-saving actions; this is called an "advance directive."

Patient Education

Equip yourself with Knowledge and Resources about your Illness and your Treatment Plan

- Ask your doctor about their special training and experience that qualifies them, or another provider to treat your illness. Google them and check out their patient recommendations. Ask them about their experience treating Black patients and their clinical outcomes. Did their Black patient do well under their care?
- Educate yourself about your illness/condition. You can obtain information from your doctor, the library, respected websites (such as the Centers for Disease Control & Prevention [CDC]), and support groups.

- Take notes during your healthcare encounter and write down important facts shared by your doctor. Ask your doctor if there are any educational resources/documents that you can take with you after the appointment or hospital visit.
- Read all medical forms and make sure you understand them before you sign anything. If you don't understand, ask your doctor or nurse to explain them.
- Make sure you know how to work any equipment that is being used in your care. If you use oxygen at home, do not smoke or let anyone smoke near you.

Tips for Staying Safe When Going to Healthcare Facilities

As Black women, we are the front lines of defense to keep our families safe from harm. It is important to remember that anytime you and your loved ones enter a healthcare facility: hospital, emergency room, doctor's office, or urgent care center, you are now at risk for contracting a deadly disease, including COVID-19. Healthcare facilities are filled with sick people, and you must protect yourself and your family. Below are tips for staying safe at any healthcare facility.

Item	Question	Tip
1	**Why are healthcare facilities dangerous?**	Hospitals, emergency rooms, and urgent care centers are filled with sick people and contagious diseases. You can contract infections during your hospital stay; they are called Hospital Acquired Infections (HAI). In addition to sick patients, many of the healthcare staff come to work while sick and spread diseases.
2	**What can I do as a patient to stay safe from COVID-19?**	You must be aware of what is needed to stay safe at a healthcare facility e.g., hospital, emergency room, or surgery center. Review the facility's pandemic safety procedures for the following: 1. Wearing a face mask when entering the facility.

Item	Question	Tip
		2. The process they use for cleaning and disinfecting the facility. 3. The type of PPE (Personal Protective Equipment) used by the care team. 4. What the care team will do to protect you and your family from the deadly coronavirus. 5. Are COVID-19 patients isolated or on the same floor with other patients. This is dangerous because you know that the virus is airborne and can travel to your hospital room. Keep your door closed and do not leave your room unless you have to.
3	**What can I do to make sure the healthcare staff follow safety procedures?**	Your safety is important, especially during the COVID-19 pandemic. Don't be afraid to ask the doctors, nurses, and other staff to wash their hands. Also, each caregiver should put on a new clean pair of gloves before touching any part of your body (drawing blood, examining your mouth, etc.). If they leave the room to get something, ask them to wash their hands and to put on a fresh pair of gloves. You do not know if they were exposed to a deadly virus when they left your

Item	Question	Tip
		room. Also, make sure that anyone who enters your room has on an approved face mask.
4	**What can I do if a healthcare worker is not following the rules?**	You have a right to a safe environment. If you are in the hospital, and a healthcare worker does not wash their hands in front of you (most rooms have hand sanitizers), ask to speak to the nurse manager or your doctor. If the explanation is that they washed their hands before they entered the room, please let them know that for your mental health, you need to watch them clean their hands.
5	**Do my visitors need to wash their hands?**	Yes. It is important for you to watch them wash their hands in front of you to keep you safe from infectious diseases.

Tips for Your Doctor's Office Appointment

As Black women, some of us may be apprehensive to be totally honest during our doctor's appointment, especially with new providers. It takes time to establish a trusting relationship with a person who is responsible for both ourselves and our families. Below is a list of tips to help you with that appointment.

Item	Question	Tip
1	**Why were you referred to this new doctor?**	As necessary, your primary care doctor may refer you to a specialist (oncologist, cardiologist, etc.) who can treat your cancer or heart disease. Please always ask the doctor why he/she is recommending you to another doctor.
2	**Why are the doctors asking personal questions?**	For the doctor to properly treat you, you must share your personal history which includes your habits. Be honest and tell the doctor if you smoke, use recreational drugs, and if you are sexually active. Please understand that your information cannot be shared without your written permission.
3	**What if I am uncomfortable sharing my medical history?**	If you are uncomfortable or possibly embarrassed, please feel free to write down your health problems and symptoms on a piece of paper. You can also take your patient advocate with you to share on your behalf.
4	**What should you ask about a new medication?**	If you are receiving a new medication, you have a right to understand the following:

Item	Question	Tip
		1. Why do you need a new medication? 2. How will the medicine help you? 3. What are the clinical outcomes for Black patients on this medication? 4. What are the names of the medicine (standard and generic)? Are generics just as effective? 5. What are the side effects? Remember the vicious cycle of healthcare shows that side effects may require new medications. 6. Can you continue to take your regular medications along with vitamins or herbal supplements? 7. Are there any foods or drinks that you should avoid when taking the new medication? 8. How long will you have to take the new medication?

Item	Question	Tip
		9. Can you get a list of all of your medications?
5	**What if the healthcare provider did not wash their hands?**	Your safety is important, especially during the COVID-19 pandemic. Don't be afraid to ask the doctors, nurses, and other staff to wash their hands. Also, each caregiver should put on a new clean pair of gloves before touching any part of your body (drawing blood, examining your mouth, body parts, etc.)
6	**What to do if you are not comfortable being alone during the exam?**	If you are anxious about being examined alone with only the doctor, let the doctor know that you want a nurse or your patient advocate to stay with you during your exam.

Tips to Improve Communication with Doctor or Provider

As Black women, some of us may be afraid to interrupt a doctor or provider to let them know that we do not understand. Perhaps they are talking or using technical terms. Use your voice and tell them that you do not understand by saying, "Excuse me. I do not understand what you are saying." Below are some helpful tips to improve your communication with your provider.

Item	Question	Tip
1	**What can you do if you don't understand your doctor?**	Healthcare providers are accountable to you. Whatever you do, please stand your ground and do not allow the provider to leave until you fully understand your healthcare diagnosis and treatment plan. Reiterate that you do not understand.
2	**What to do if the doctor is rushing?**	Ask the doctor if you need to schedule another appointment when they are available to answer your questions.
3	**What can you do if you have trouble reading or cannot read?**	Don't be embarrassed if you have problems reading medical information. Tell your caregivers and they can help explain your medical documents and educational materials.

Item	Question	Tip
4	**What to do if you do not understand how to take your medications?**	Some patients don't understand how to take their medication. If a patient takes too much or too little of the medicine, this can be dangerous. Tell your doctor if you need help with when and how to take your medications.
5	**What if you can't remember all of your medical information?**	Ask your doctor if they have a card with all of your medications and the times that you must take your medication. Then, take the card with you to every doctor's appointment.
6	**Why do I need to sign an informed consent?**	If you need to have a procedure or surgery, you will need to sign an informed consent. This document is required by law and means that you: 1. Understand your illness or condition. 2. Understand how your illness will be treated. 3. You agree on the treatment plan including surgery. 4. You understand the risks of the treatment. 5. You understand the risks if you are not treated.

Item	Question	Tip
		6. You will need to decide if you will sign the paperwork only after the consent was explained to you. Ask questions if you do not thoroughly understand the informed consent document.
7	**What to do if the doctor's instructions are not clear?**	Ask the doctor to write down the instructions if the oral instructions are not clear. Also, ask them to tell your patient advocate the instructions.
8	**How can you remember how and when to take your medications?**	Some doctors have medication cards. Ask your doctor to fill out your medication card. Always keep the card with you.

Tips for a Crucial Conversation

As Black women, we are sometimes invisible as we navigate the complex healthcare system. Perhaps a doctor was abrupt about explaining your diagnosis and treatment plan, or you feel that your voice is not being heard. You can request a consult or an appointment with your doctor. Use the tips below to prepare for your crucial conversation.

Item	Question	Tip
1	**How should you prepare for the conversation?**	1. Do your homework. Before your meeting with the doctor, be prepared by learning about your disease or the proposed intervention so that you feel empowered with your decisions. 2. List what you want to discuss. 3. Write down your goal for the conversation. 4. Be prepared to share your feelings of marginalization, disrespect, being ignored, or intimidation. Remember, no one can tell you how you feel. 5. Be open to the doctor's perspective as to why he was abrupt or failed to communicate more clearly. After all, anyone can have a bad day and be overwhelmed.

Item	Question	Tip
		6. Remain positive that you will have a productive conversation with good outcomes. 7. Practice what you will say with a family member or friend to reduce any anxieties.
2	**What to do during the conversation?**	1. Stay calm, cool, and collected during the conversation since it is about your health and good clinical outcomes. 2. Be comfortable and confident that you can have this conversation and achieve positive results. 3. Remember that the doctor is not above you, and that you are equal. 4. Acknowledge that you are not a healthcare expert, but you are the expert on your body and life experience.

Item	Question	Tip
		5. Take notes during the conversation so that you do not forget anything important. 6. Do not end the conversation until you are satisfied that all of your concerns have been addressed.
3	**What to do after the conversation?**	1. You can document your conversation with either a letter or even an email that captures the conversation. The letter or email should include your understanding of what you both agreed on regarding your healthcare. 2. If you feel that you did not get your desired outcome, you can explore other options, including a formal complaint.
4	**How to write a complaint regarding your healthcare?**	1. If you feel that your crucial conversation did not end well, you can write a letter to document your concerns. 2. The letter is your next step that will not only document your concerns but also inform patient relations of the issue.

Tips for Writing a Complaint about Your Healthcare

Black women are often labeled with the racist trope, "Angry Black Woman." It is so crucial for you to find your voice and formally complain about healthcare problems with either care delivery or your treatment. Below are tips for writing your complaint to a healthcare provider, or the hospital's patient relations department. This is the department that will investigate your complaint. Check the hospital's website for their address, contact number, and email. You can call the department to see "who" to send your letter to and what you want in the form of service recovery.

Item	Question	Tip
1	**What to include in your complaint letter?**	1. Include your name and address as the complainant. 2. Include the date of the treatment or incident and the person(s) who was involved in the care delivery. 3. Provide a brief description of what happened. 4. State your expected action and possible outcomes. 5. Include any copies of supporting documentation.

2	**Who to send your complaint to?**	A complaint letter to a hospital may be addressed directly to the following: 1. Doctor that was responsible for poor care delivery that cause your dissatisfaction. 2. Nurse that was responsible for poor care delivery that caused your dissatisfaction. 3. Other staff that was responsible for poor care delivery that caused your dissatisfaction. 4. Head of the department, for example emergency room. 5. Head of the nursing unit. 6. Head of patient relations department (see hospital website for the name and phone number). 7. Head of the hospital, the Board of Health or another regulatory agency.
3	**What to expect after your complaint letter?**	1. You should receive a letter from the patient relations department acknowledging receipt of your complaint and detailing the next steps.

		2. If you do not receive a letter from the patient relations department contact them by phone.
4	**What to do if you do not hear from the hospital Patient Relations Department or their resolution is not appropriate?**	If you still are not satisfied with the response, you can take additional action by issuing a formal complaint to one or more of the following: 1. The Joint Commission (Regulatory Agency) 2. State Health Agency and your State Representative 3. Board of Health You can also contact an attorney and take legal action for any harm that you suffered from medical negligence.

Sample Complaint Letter to a Hospital

Patient's Name
Patient's Address
City, State, Zip Code
Phone number

Date

Name of Contact Person from the Patient Relations Department
Name of Hospital
Hospital Address
City, State, Zip Code

Re: Emergency Room Quality of Care

Dear Mr / Ms Name of Person,

On January 27, 2022, I entered your emergency room for treatment of my swollen ankle. I waited for four hours in excruciating pain before being admitted into the examining room. I waited another 45 minutes and was finally seen by Doctor Name and Nurse Name. An X-ray was taken, and I waited another two hours. Finally, I was seen by the doctor and was told that there was no issue and told to take aspirin for pain.

Since the pain did not subside after two days, I went to Name of other Hospital, where an X-ray was taken that showed my ankle was fractured.

Since I suffered unnecessarily, I would like to know that the doctor and nurse who attended to me in your hospital have been reprimanded for this negligence. Enclosed are copies of the documents from the second hospital.

I know the emergency room was very crowded, but when I finally saw a doctor, I expected an accurate diagnosis.

Kindly let me know what, if any, action will be taken in this case. I am home every day and can be reached at 555 123 4567 or name@email.com.

Sincerely,

Patient's signature
Patient's name
List of enclosures

Tips to Ensure a Safe Surgery or Procedure

As Black women, we may have heard the horror stories of how we are treated in the operating room, while sedated and not able to voice our concerns. It broke my heart when I saw the video of the Black woman who secretly recorded her surgery and later listened to the disgusting comments made about her during the surgery. Hopefully, in the near future, a video of each surgery will become a part of the medical record. Until that happens, please review the tips below to ensure a safe surgery (hip replacement) or a procedure (colonoscopy).

Item	Question	Tip
1	**What should you ask your surgeon before your scheduled surgery or procedure?**	Be aware that a safe surgery actually begins in what you do to prepare for your surgery. Make sure that you review the following with your surgeon and their staff: 1. Your current medications and if and when you have to stop taking them. 2. When to stop eating and drinking before your surgery. 3. Your options for anesthesia or sedation. 4. Your pain management plan, yes Black people do feel pain. 5. Your surgeon's clinical outcomes for Black patients for

Item	Question	Tip
		your specific surgery. E.g., for a knee replacement, ask what percentage of Black patients return to normal daily activities? 6. Review all surgical documents including your advance directives and the naming of your healthcare proxy.
2	**What to do the day before and on the day of surgery or procedure?**	1. Do not eat or drink if told not to (you may stop the day before your surgery). 2. Do not wear nail polish – your nails show if you are getting oxygen during the surgery. 3. Do not wear makeup – your natural face color will help to show if your blood is circulating properly. 4. Identify who will drive home if you are leaving the same day of your surgery or procedure.
3	**What will happen before**	Before your surgery, you will have an assessment by the care team and it will include: 1. Confirmation of signed Informed Consent form

Item	Question	Tip
	your surgery or procedure?	2. Confirmation of your type of surgery and the exact location (for example "right" knee replacement surgery) 3. Your limb or body part will be "marked" by a caregiver, please speak up if the location is incorrect. 4. If you are having surgery that requires imaging, check to ensure that the surgeon has the correct images. 5. Confirmation that you have discussed the risks of the surgery with your doctor. 6. Discuss the type of implants or medical devices that you may get during the surgery. 7. Discuss what is included in your post-surgical care plan. Ask your surgeon about how to care for your incisions and if you will have any drains or lines after surgery. 8. Ask your surgeon if the surgical team follows the Universal Protocol, which requires the team to take a "time out" before the surgery starts. This is to make

Item	Question	Tip
		sure that the team knows that you are the correct patient for the surgery that is scheduled.
4	**What will happen after your surgery?**	1. Surgery requires an incision and that means pain. It is important to let your doctor or nurse if you are in pain. 2. If you are to receive a new medication, find out the reason and possible side effects. Tell the team if you have any allergies to medications before they are ordered. E.g., some patients may be allergic to penicillin. 3. Check the status of your intravenous (IV) fluids that allow medications and fluids to be administered to your vein. Find out how long it should take for the bag to be emptied and tell the nurse if the IV drip is either too fast or too slow. 4. Notify the nurse that you may have an infection based on the following: • Fever, chills, or fatigue. • Swelling, redness, or pain around your surgical incision site.

Item	Question	Tip
		• Any discoloration of the fluid from your surgical wound. 5. Before you are discharged, make sure that you schedule your follow-up appointment, get your prescriptions, and review the instructions of your discharge plan.
5	**What is needed to stay safe during the COVID-19 and I have to have surgery?**	It is urgent that you are aware of what is needed to stay safe at the facility (hospital or surgery center). Review the facility's pandemic safety procedures for the following: 1. Wearing a face mask when entering the facility. 2. The process for cleaning and disinfecting the facility. 3. The type of PPE (Personal Protective Equipment) used by the care team. 4. What the care team will do to protect you and your family from the deadly coronavirus. 5. What actions you must take if you develop fever or cold symptoms the day before your surgery.

Tips for a Safe Hospital Discharge and No Readmission

As Black women, we may not be aware that Black patients have a higher readmission rate to the hospital within 30 days of discharge compared to white patients. As a healthcare consultant, I learned that many hospitals assign a "Readmission Risk Score" to each patient that should improve during the hospital visit. For example, if you were admitted to the hospital for the problem of "shortness of breath." A proper diagnosis and treatment plan should resolve the problem and reduce the risk prior to discharge. In addition, if you are at high risk for readmission, you should expect to receive early intervention upon discharge to make sure that you do not have to return to the hospital for the same problem. Remember with the COVID-19 pandemic, a hospital is a dangerous place and you do not want to be admitted to the hospital unnecessarily. Please review the tips below on how to have a safe hospital discharge and avoid a return trip to the hospital.

Item	Question	Tip
1	**What is a safe hospital discharge?**	It is your right to leave the hospital whenever you want before you are officially discharged. However, it is important to know that you are not a prisoner. This is called an AMA (Against Medical Advice). You can also request to be transferred to another healthcare institution. This will require a transfer and handoff between both facilities. A safe discharge is when the doctor writes your discharge order with instructions and ensures

		that you are ready to leave the hospital. If you feel that you are not ready to leave due to your health, voice your concerns. The discharge instructions will include: 1. Your prognosis and treatment 2. Your medication 3. Your need for outpatient services 4. Your follow-up care
2	**What to ask while you are still in the hospital** **Plan your discharge**	It is important for you to plan for your discharge. During your hospital visit, your plan of care (POC) is reviewed by your care team every day and they will have an estimate of your discharge date. While planning for your discharge, ask the following and make sure that you take notes to record their responses. 1. What was the final diagnosis? 2. Is it a new condition? 3. Is a follow-up appointment needed? 4. What medications have been prescribed? 5. What should I do when I get home? 6. Do I need to have someone with me at home?

		7. When can I return to work? 8. Who do I call if I have any problems? Don't forget to arrange for someone to pick you up from the hospital and take you home.

Tips for Your Day of Discharge from the Hospital

Item	Question	Tip
1	**What to ask the day of your discharge?** **Day of Discharge**	You will be informed of your discharge typically the day before. However, due to COVID-19, you may be informed on the same day. A nurse will review your discharge instructions with you and your patient advocate (family). Take notes regarding the following questions. 1. What is the likelihood that I will be readmitted? 2. What is my readmission risk rating (high, medium, or low)? 3. If you are at a medium or high risk of readmission, what actions will be taken to reduce your risk. E.g., a phone call from a nurse to check on your aftercare or discharge with home care services, or an appointment with your primary care provider to examine you. 4. Do I have any physical limitations? E.g., no stairs, no heavy lifting, or bed rest only. 5. Do I have to avoid anything: food, caffeine, alcohol, tobacco, recreational drugs, vitamins, or supplements?

		6. Do I need any referrals from the following: • New doctors including Specialists • Tests, home care, or therapy (physical or occupational) • Any medical equipment (e.g., oxygen tank, wheelchair)
2	**Should I take notes?**	Yes. Buy a small notebook and keep it with you during your hospital visit. During the day of discharge record the responses to your questions. 1. Ask for clarification if you don't understand something and write down the response. 2. Write down the dates of any scheduled follow-up appointments or therapy. 3. Write down the names, doses, and frequency for any new medications.

		4. Write down the names of who you should contact if you have any problems at home with your health. For example, if you are having problems with your oxygen machine, who do you contact?

Tips for Obtaining a Second Opinion

As Black women, we must use our voice and seek a second opinion regarding our healthcare needs. For example, research shows that white doctors do not enroll Black patients in healthcare programs or at the same rate as white patients due to racial bias. This can be harmful to our health. It is always important for us to find our voice and seek other providers for a second opinion to offer input and advice.

Item	Question	Tip
1	**What is a second opinion?**	As a patient, if your doctor informs you of a diagnosis and treatment (medical intervention), you have the right to contact another doctor for their opinion. In some cases, time is of the essence, for example a stage 4 cancer diagnosis will require urgent action for a second opinion.
2	**Why should you get a second opinion?**	Your reasons for getting a second opinion are personal, and you do not need to feel guilty for obtaining additional health information about your disease and treatment options. 1. You do not feel comfortable with how you were treated during the consult. 2. The surgeon does not have a good reputation. 3. Your gut tells you that something is not right.

		4. You want to empower yourself and talk to at least one other doctor about your case.
3	**What are the benefits of getting a second opinion?**	The are many benefits to getting a second opinion as noted below: 1. Confirmation – You may want another doctor to review your case to confirm the first diagnosis which may give you peace of mind. 2. Help with your decision – You may want to explore your options and getting a second opinion may offer new information about your disease. 3. Different medical backgrounds – Not all doctors think exactly alike, thus a fresh assessment of your medical condition may provide a different approach to your treatment.

Tips for Using the Patient Portal to Obtain Your Health Records

As Black women, we know that knowledge is power. Thereby, review your health records that are available online via the Hospitals' Patient Portal. It is a federal law, via the Affordable Care Act that all patients have access to their medical health records. You can obtain a hard copy of your medical records by contacting the provider and they will be mailed to you within 30 days. However, if you want to see your medical records immediately, you can access them via the Patient Portal.

Item	Question	Tip
1	**What is the Patient Portal?**	A Patient Portal is essentially a personal website for your healthcare. Only you and to those you give permission can see your medical records. The portal is convenient and allows 24-hour access. Many patient portals allow you to schedule appointments and send emails to your providers.
2	**How do I access the Patient Portal?**	You can contact your provider or hospital to find out how to access the Patient Portal. Many healthcare providers will email you the link to access the Patient Portal or the phone number to call if you need help accessing your Patient Portal.

3	**What information can be seen on the Patient Portal?**	The Patient Portal is a great tool to help you keep track of your healthcare information including: 1. Recent doctor visits 2. Recent emergency room visits 3. Discharge summaries 4. Clinical progress notes 5. Medications 6. Immunizations 7. Allergies 8. Laboratory results
4	**What information is not available on the Patient Portal?**	The Patient Portal does not have sensitive healthcare information. The following is not available on the Patient Portal. 1. Behavioral health records 2. Protected minor children visits 3. Business records 4. Research data if you were in a clinical trial

5	**What are the benefits of the Patient Portal?**	The main benefit is improved communication between the patient and provider. This should not only improve your patient experience but also improve your relationship with your provider.
6	**What can I do if there is an error on my medical record?**	If you find an error on your patient record, for example, lab results that do not belong to you (it happens due to the same names or similar names), contact the Patient Portal Helpline and inform them of the errors. You do not want medical errors on your patient records.

STOP Tool: How to Take a Breath

As Black women, we are overwhelmed with myriad daily responsibilities. We work, we raise children, and sometimes husbands. We take care of our elderly parents and are often the backbone of the entire family. I created that STOP tool for you to use during your healthcare encounters. The STOP tool is a quick reminder of what to do before beginning any healthcare visit. STOP and be mindful of what you are experiencing and be aware of how you are being treated.

You are an advocate for your health - STOP and be mindful of what is going on before you begin your visit to the Healthcare facility for services.

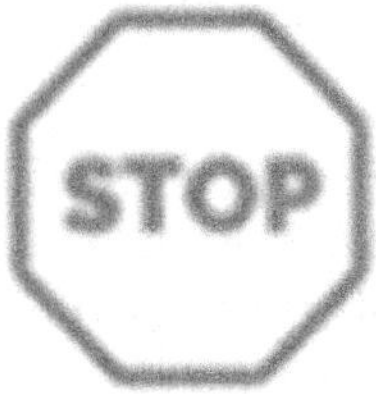

Stop. Before you go to your healthcare visit including appointments and emergency room, stop and check to see what you need to take with you. Make sure that you have a pen and paper to take down the names and information that you need or use your cell phone to capture and record your healthcare experience.

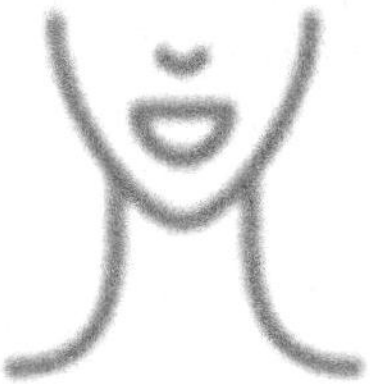

Take a Breath. Whenever you are having a healthcare crisis, it is important to take a breath. Tell yourself to be mindful. Be aware of what is happening to you or your family member or friend. Remember that you are valued and your life matters. You deserve to be treated with respect and dignity.

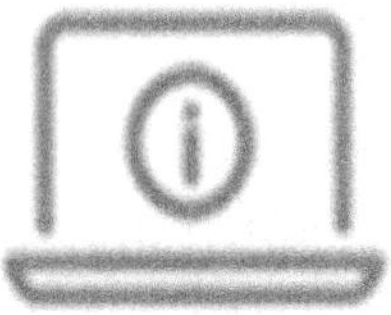

Observe. Be aware of what is going on during your healthcare visit. Observe who is providing the care and ask for information. Use your cell phone if available to "Google" information that you do not understand. Don't forget that you have a patient's right to understand your diagnosis and proposed intervention.

Preparedness. Are you prepared mentally to go to your healthcare visit? Do you have your checklists for you visit? Do you have a patient advocate to attend your visit with you? Always ask a family member or friend to be your advocate, especially during a healthcare crisis.

CONCLUSION

The vicissitudes of life often force one to ask the question, "How did I get here?" For me, as a Black healthcare consultant and engineer in the United States of America, I have often pondered myriad questions about Black healthcare in America including: Why was I sent home from the hospital to die with a ruptured appendix? Was this the standard practice for Black patients? Why do Black people have the highest rate of not only acquiring but also dying from chronic diseases including high blood pressure, diabetes, kidney disease, and cancer? Why do Black women have the highest rate of maternal mortality? Why do Black babies die at a rate eight times higher than white babies? Why do Black people have the highest death rate for the new global pandemic, coronavirus SARS2 or COVID-19? The common denominator as I sought answers to those queries was white supremacy racism. I wrote this book to help Black women understand the impact of white supremacy racism in healthcare and to create a patient advocate toolkit for Black survival.

Until recently, the explanation for the horrific health disparities in America was often flippantly stated as poverty which for centuries was simply a euphemism for Black people. Just blame the victim themselves for their own pathology. However, in the 1960s with the Civil Rights laws in place that allowed the formation of a Black middle class, when analyzing healthcare data by class, it was clear that regardless of economic status, Black people still had worse clinical outcomes. The reason was systemic or institutional racism. In order for Black people to win at healthcare, a patient toolkit is essential. This toolkit will provide you with the knowledge and skills to be prepared for any healthcare scenario that makes you feel disrespected or devalued. It is important for you to understand this is how racism is embedded in healthcare so that you can protect yourself and your family. You are not going crazy when a healthcare provider assumes that as a Black woman you are a single mother. You are not going crazy when you tell a healthcare provider that you are in pain and you are not offered pain medication because the historic belief as taught in medical schools is that Black people have a higher pain tolerance than white people, thus pain medication is not readily prescribed.[27]

Since the May 25th, 2020 murder of George Floyd, a black man who was murdered by Derek Chauvin, a white Minneapolis police officer after the report of using a fake twenty-dollar bill at a corner store, there was a series of actions by white institutions across America. It was a short period of what some have labeled, "racial reckoning in America." Unfortunately, these actions do not include a national apology for "slavery" or trillions of dollars for reparations for four centuries of lost wealth due to unpaid Black labor.

The reckoning consisted of myriad businesses, local governments, and even healthcare institutions, sharing their new commitment to antiracism and apologies for past misbehaviors. Countless businesses also donated to Black institutions to support racial justice and equity. There were two institutions that caught my attention that were featured on several social media platforms. The first news feed from the Centers for Disease Control (CDC). The CDC leadership was in the news daily to provide national COVID-19 updates. It was the CDC that shared the news of how the deadly virus had not only infected Black people at a higher rate than white people but that Black people also had the highest rate of death upon contracting COVID-19. So, it was a pleasant surprise when the following occurred in 2021. Two declarations by the CDC and the APA were quite intriguing in that they committed to future actions to address and repair past misdeeds The CDC declared racism as a public health crisis and the APA apologized for using racist practices for decades to the detriment of Black psychological health. It is those actions that I include in the book with the hope to understand what actions and behaviors are needed by white people to address past harm.

Instead of waiting with bated breath for white controlled healthcare institutions to treat all customers equitably, I decided to share my healthcare consulting knowledge with Black women. During my career, I conducted endless Voice of the Customer (VOC) surveys to find out what patients and family members value in the healthcare experience. I was not surprised that 100% of survey participants agreed that a patient toolkit would be beneficial. This book and toolkit provide information to help you understand your rights as a patient, and what to expect during healthcare visits at emergency rooms, hospitals, and doctor's offices.

This book and toolkit also help provide information on how to "Voice Your Concerns" to ensure that you are safe throughout the healthcare encounter. I personally had to learn how to use my voice and speak up during my own healthcare emergency. In retrospect, if I had a toolkit, I would not have waited until my third emergency room visit to take action to save my own life. I could have avoided weeks of pain and suffering. In retrospect, I was able to take a very careful and comprehensive look and evaluate what actually happened to me including being sent home with acute appendicitis and antibiotics after my first emergency room visit, to then return and be sent home a second time with a ruptured appendix, albeit this time with intravenous antibiotics. It wasn't until my third emergency room visit, that God gave me my voice to demand the healthcare that I needed to save my life. It is with my deepest desire that I share what I know as a healthcare consultant for you to learn, understand, and be empowered to save your life and those that you love. May God forever bless you and yours.

REFERENCES

1. Published: Feb 25, 2022. (2022, February 25). Global Covid-19 tracker – updated as of February 25. KFF. Retrieved February 26, 2022, from https://www.kff.org/coronavirus-covid-19/issue-brief/global-covid-19-tracker
2. Centers for Disease Control and Prevention. (2022, February 25). CDC Covid Data tracker. Centers for Disease Control and Prevention. Retrieved February 26, 2022, from https://covid.cdc.gov/covid-data-tracker/#demographics
3. Eligon, J. (2020, December 24). Black doctor dies of Covid-19 after complaining of racist treatment. The New York Times. Retrieved November 1, 2021, from https://www.nytimes.com/2020/12/23/us/susan-moore-black-doctor-indiana.html
4. Hutchinson, B. (2020, November 30). ABC News. Retrieved November 1, 2021, from https://abcnews.go.com/US/hospital-ceos-response-black-doctors-covid-19-death/story?id=74971005
5. Directly addressing the issue of racial equity in our facilities. IU Health. (2020, December 24). Retrieved November 1, 2021, from https://iuhealth.org/for-media/press-releases/directly-addressing-the-issue-of-racial-equity-in-our-facilities

6. Williams, S. (2022, April 5). How Serena Williams saved her own life. *Elle*. Retrieved April 16, 2022, from https://www.elle.com/life-love/a39586444/how-serena-williams-saved-her-own-life/

7. About us - history: Pittsburgh, PA. Primary Care Health Services, Inc. (n.d.). Retrieved November 1, 2021, from http://pchspitt.org/about-us/history (Alma Illery Medical Center History)

8. Pitt Swanson School of Engineering. (2020, October 20). Pitt Engineering alumnus dedicates major gift toward undergraduate tuition support. Retrieved November 1, 2021, from https://news.engineering.pitt.edu/pitt-engineering-alumnus-dedicates-major-gift-toward-undergraduate-tuition-support/

9. Johnson, R. (2020, August 26). 'Embarrassing': Black Student Leaders Criticize Low Black student enrollment. The Pitt News. Retrieved November 1, 2021, from https://pittnews.com/article/159455/featured/embarrassing-black-student-leaders-criticize-low-black-student-enrollment/

10. DeSilver, D. (2020, August 27). Black unemployment rate is consistently twice that of whites. Pew Research Center. Retrieved November 1, 2021, from https://www.pewresearch.org/fact-tank/2013/08/21/through-good-times-and-bad-black-unemployment-is-consistently-double-that-of-whites/

11. https://www.pewresearch.org/2010/12/14/reagans-recession/

12. Identical Twins Tell How They Differ. (1992, March 9). *Jet* Magazine, 81(20), 34–37.

13. New York: Harper & Row. King, Martin Luther, 1929-1968, Where Do We Go from Here: Chaos or Community? New York: Harper & Row, 1967.

14. Di Angelo, Robin, 1956, *White Fragility, Why Is It So Hard for White People to Talk About Racism*, Beacon Press, 2020.

15. Cress Welsing, Frances, *The Isis Papers, The Keys to the Colors*, Chicago, Third World, Press, 1991.

16. Encyclopedia Britannica, inc. *Britannica Dictionary definition of the word, race.* Encyclopedia Britannica. Retrieved April 16, 2022, from https://www.britannica.com/dictionary/race

17. Black Hospitals in the United States, Encyclopedia of African-American Culture and History. Retrieved November 1, 2021, from Encyclopedia.com https://www.encyclopedia.com/history/encyclopedias-almanacs-transcripts-and-maps/hospitals-united-states-black

18. Ault, A. (2021, April 19) Percentage of Doctors Who Are Black Barely Changed in 120 Years. Retrieved November 1, 2021, from https://www.medscape.com/viewarticle/949673#:~:text=In%201940%2C%202.8%25%20of%20physicians,Journal%20of%20General%20Internal%20Medicine.

19. Hannah-Jones, N., Roper, C., Silverman, I., & Silverstein, J. (2022). The 1619 project: A new origin story. Random House Large Print, a division of Penguin Random House LLC.

20. John Punch Decision, July 9, 1640. Retrieved November 1, 2021, from https://www.law.berkeley.edu/library/legal-research/black-americans-and-the-law/

21. Slave. Definition, Oxford Advanced Learner's Dictionary at OxfordLearnersDictionaries.com. (n.d.). Retrieved November 1, 2021, from https://www.oxfordlearnersdictionaries.com/us/definition/english/slave_1#:~:text=slave-,noun,work%20for%20and%20obey%20them

22. Telling the Story, Enslavement of African People in the United States. Retrieved November 1, 2021, from https://www.buffalolib.org/sites/default/files/exhibit/pdf/Vocab%20&%20Key%20Concepts%20-%20mc.pdf

23. Byrd, W. M., & Clayton, L. A. (2001, March). Race, Medicine, and Health Care in the United States: A Historical Survey. Journal of the National Medical Association. Retrieved November 1, 2021, from https://www.ncbi.nlm.nih.gov/pmc/articles/PMC2593958/

24. 15th amendment to the U.S. Constitution: Primary Documents in American history: Introduction. Research Guides. (n.d.). Retrieved April 16, 2022, from https://guides.loc.gov/15th-amendment

25. Berlin, Ira, *Remembering Slavery: African Americans Talk About Their Personal Experiences of Slavery and Emancipation*, New Press, New York, Library of Congress, Washington, D.C. 1998.

26. Kyere, Eric, Enslaved people's health was ignored from the country's beginning, laying the groundwork for today's health disparities, July 30, 2020. Retrieved November 1, 2021, from https://theconversation.com/enslaved-peoples-health-was-ignored-from-the-countrys-beginning-laying-the-groundwork-for-todays-health-disparities-143339

27. Anderson, Claude, *Black Labor, White Wealth: The Search for Power and Economic Justice*, Bethesda, Maryland: PowerNomics Corporation of America, 1994.

28. Hoffman, K., Racial Bias in Pain Assessment and Treatment Recommendations, and Raise Beliefs About Biological Differences Between Blacks and Whites. Procedures National Academy Sciences USA. 2016 Apr 19; 113(16): 4296–4301. Retrieved November 1, 2021, from https://www.ncbi.nlm.nih.gov/pmc/articles/PMC4843483/

29. DeGruy, Joy, *Post Traumatic Slave Syndrome: America's Legacy of Enduring Injury and Healing*, Joy DeGruy Publications, Inc., September 11, 2017.

30. Benjamin, George C., *Health Inequity from the Founding of the Freedmen's Bureau to COVID-19*, AMA Journal of Ethics, February, 2021.

31. Bennett, Lerone, Jr., 1928-2018. *Before the Mayflower; a History of the Negro in America, 1619-1964*. Baltimore: Penguin Books, 19681964.

32. Slave Law in Colonial Virginia: A Timeline. Retrieved November 1, 2021, from https://www.shsu.edu/~jll004/vabeachcourse_spring09/bacons_rebellion/slavelawincolonialvirginiatimeline.pdf

33. United States Congress. "The Civil Rights Act of 1866". Law, April 09, 1866. Teaching American History. Retrieved November 1, 2021, from https://teachingamericanhistory.org/document/the-civil-rights-act-of-1866/

34. FDR signs Social Security Act, History.com Editors. Retrieved November 1, 2021, from https://www.history.com/this-day-in-history/fdr-signs-social-security-act, Accessed 10/12/2021.

35. *Failing Economy, Failing Health*. Harvard Public Health Magazine. (2019, January 15). Retrieved November 1, 2021, from https://www.hsph.harvard.edu/magazine/magazine_article/failing-economy-failing-health/

36. Rook, D. A brief history of employer-sponsored healthcare [from the 1930s to now]. Retrieved October 28, 2021, from https://www.griffinbenefits.com/blog/history-of-employer-sponsored-healthcare

37. A brief history: Universal health care efforts in the US. (2021, May 03). Retrieved November 1, 2021, from https://pnhp.org/a-brief-history-universal-health-care-efforts-in-the-us/

38. Herzlinger, R. (2020, December 9). Give employees cash to purchase their own insurance. Harvard Business Review. Retrieved November 1, 2021, from https://hbr.org/2020/12/give-employees-cash-to-purchase-their-own-insurance

39. Garfield, Rachel (2020, May 13). The uninsured and the ACA: A primer – key facts about health insurance and the uninsured amidst changes to the Affordable Care Act - how many people are uninsured? KFF. Retrieved November 1, 2021, from https://www.kff.org/report-section/the-uninsured-and-the-aca-a-primer-key-facts-about-health-insurance-and-the-uninsured-amidst-changes-to-the-affordable-care-act-how-many-people-are-uninsured/

40. Press, A. (2017, January 20). GOP governors who turned down Medicaid money have hands out. Modern Healthcare. Retrieved November 1, 2021, from https://www.modernhealthcare.com/article/20170119/NEWS/170119871/gop-governors-who-turned-down-medicaid-money-have-hands-out

41. Laguipo, A. B. B. (2021, June 22). Study shows that covid-19 was present in five U.S. states in December 2019, even before the first reported case in China. News. Retrieved November 1, 2021, from https://www.news-medical.net/news/20210621/Study-shows-that-COVID-19-was-present-in-five-states-in-December-2019-even-before-the-first-reported-case-in-China.aspx

42. Peters, C. (2020, June 8). A detailed timeline of all the ways Trump failed to respond to the coronavirus. Vox. Retrieved November 1, 2021, from https://www.vox.com/2020/6/8/21242003/trump-failed-coronavirus-response

43. Evans, M. (2015, February 21). Hospitals face closures as 'a new day in Healthcare' dawns. Modern Healthcare. Retrieved November 1, 2021, from https://www.modernhealthcare.com/article/20150221/MAGAZINE/302219988/hospitals-face-closures-as-a-new-day-in-healthcare-dawns

44. Aacharya, R. P., & Gastmans, C. (2011). Emergency department triage: An ethical analysis. BMC Emergency Medicine, 11(1), 1–12. https://doi.org/10.1186/1471-227x-11-16

45. Roberts, J. (2020, November 16). What is triage and why is it important? NHS GP Practices: Econsult Blog. eConsult. Retrieved November 1, 2021, from https://econsult.net/blog/what-is-triage

46. Emergency severity index (ESI): A triage tool for emergency department. AHRQ. (2012, September). Retrieved November 1, 2021, from https://www.ahrq.gov/patient-safety/settings/emergency-dept/esi.html

47. Cairns, C. (2021, February 19). Emergency Department Visits by Selected Characteristics 2018. Centers for Disease Control and Prevention. Retrieved November 1, 2021, from https://www.cdc.gov/nchs/products/databriefs/db401.htm

48. Emergency severity index (ESI): A triage tool for emergency department. AHRQ. (2012, September). Retrieved November 1, 2021, from https://www.ahrq.gov/patient-safety/settings/emergency-dept/esi.html

49. Grubbs, V. (2021, June 23). *The Health Care System has the Black Community in a Choke Hold*. California Health Care Foundation. Retrieved February 13, 2022, from https://www.chcf.org/blog/health-care-system-has-black-community-choke-hold/

50. 2018 percentage of active US physicians Figure 18. percentage of all active physicians by Race/ethnicity, 2018. AAMC. (n.d.). Retrieved November 1, 2021, from https://www.aamc.org/data-reports/workforce/interactive-data/figure-18-percentage-all-active-physicians-race/ethnicity-2018

51. American Psychological Association. (n.d.). APA Dictionary of Psychology. American Psychological Association. Retrieved November 1, 2021, from https://dictionary.apa.org/intergenerational-trauma

52. American Psychological Association, (2021, October 29), Apology to People of Color for APA's Role in Promoting, Perpetuating, and Failing to Challenge Racism, Racial Discrimination, and Human Hierarchy in U.S. Retrieved November 1, 2021, from https://www.apa.org/about/policy/racism-apology

53. American Psychological Association. (n.d.). Role of psychology and APA in dismantling systemic racism in U.S. American Psychological Association. Retrieved November 1, 2021, from https://www.apa.org/about/policy/dismantling-systemic-racism

54. Centers for Disease Control and Prevention. (2021, November 24). Racism and health. Centers for Disease Control and Prevention. Retrieved February 1, 2022, from https://www.cdc.gov/coronavirus/2019-ncov/community/health-equity/race-ethnicity.html

55. Leonard, J. (2021, May 16). What is health inequity? definition, examples, and root causes. Medical News Today. Retrieved November 1, 2021, from https://www.medicalnewstoday.com/articles/health-inequity

56. 2020 Census - Pew Research Center. (2021, September 30). Behind Biden's 2020 victory. Pew Research Center - U.S. Politics & Policy. Retrieved November 1, 2021, from https://www.pewresearch.org/politics/2021/06/30/behind-bidens-2020-victory/

57. Pew vote 2012- How the faithful voted: 2012 preliminary analysis. Pew Research Center's Religion & Public Life Project. (2020, May 30). Retrieved November 1, 2021, from https://www.pewforum.org/2012/11/07/how-the-faithful-voted-2012-preliminary-exit-poll-analysis/

58. Black Funding Denied: Community Foundation support for Black Communities. National Committee for Responsive Philanthropy. (2021, June 16). Retrieved November 1, 2021, from https://www.ncrp.org/2020/08/black-funding-denied.html

59. Christian, M. (2008, May 26). Kemba Smith Teaches the Importance of Making the Right Decisions. *Jet Magazine*, 56–58.

60. National Institute on Drug Abuse. (2022, January 19). Words matter - terms to use and avoid when talking about addiction. National Institute on Drug Abuse. Retrieved January 30, 2022, from https://www.drugabuse.gov/nidamed-medical-health-professionals/health-professions-education/words-matter-terms-to-use-avoid-when-talking-about-addiction

61. Dugan, K. T. (2021, July 20). What you should know about Jeff Bezos' Tuesday space launch. *Fortune*. Retrieved November 1, 2021, from https://fortune.com/2021/07/19/jeff-bezos-space-launch-blue-origin-july-20-2021-billionaires/

62. Better use of money - McCarthy, J. (2021, July 20). Jeff Bezos just spent $5.5B to be in space for 4 minutes. here are 7 things that money could help solve. Global Citizen. Retrieved November 1, 2021, from https://www.globalcitizen.org/en/content/jeff-bezos-space-flight-money-better-uses/

63. Published by Statista Research Department. (2021, September 21). U.S. Poverty Rate, by Ethnicity 2020. Statista. Retrieved November 1, 2021, from https://www.statista.com/statistics/200476/us-poverty-rate-by-ethnic-group/

64. CARES Act - Treasury and IRS announce families of nearly 60 million children receive $15 billion in first payments of expanded and newly advanceable child tax credit. U.S. Department of the Treasury. (2021, August 3). Retrieved November 1, 2021, from https://home.treasury.gov/news/press-releases/Treasury-and-IRS-Announce-Families-of-Nearly-60-Million-Children-Receive-%2415-Billion-Dollars-in-First-Payments-of-Expanded-and-Newly-Advanceable-Child-Tax-Credit

65. Reeves, R. V. (2021, March 11). New Child Tax Credit could slash poverty now and boost social mobility later. Brookings. Retrieved November 1, 2021, from https://www.brookings.edu/blog/up-front/2021/03/11/new-child-tax-credit-could-slash-poverty-now-and-boost-social-mobility-later/

66. Broady, K. E., & Barr, A. (2021, December 6). Despite a strong October jobs report, black unemployment remains too high to justify the Fed's recent decision to decrease bond purchases. Brookings. Retrieved October 1, 2021, from https://www.brookings.edu/blog/the-avenue/2021/11/08/despite-a-strong-october-jobs-report-black-unemployment-remains-too-high-to-justify-the-feds-recent-decision-to-decrease-bond-purchases/

67. Childress, S. (2014, May 15). Report: School segregation is back, 60 years after "Brown". PBS. Retrieved November 1, 2021, from https://www.pbs.org/wgbh/frontline/article/report-school-segregation-is-back-60-years-after-brown/

68. Rivkin, S. (2020, August 5). Desegregation since the Coleman Report. Education Next. Retrieved November 1, 2021, from https://www.educationnext.org/desegregation-since-the-coleman-report-racial-composition-student-learning/

69. Finnegold, K. (2021, February 11). HP-2021-02 trends in the U.S. uninsured population, 2010-2020. Retrieved November 1, 2021, from https://aspe.hhs.gov/sites/default/files/private/pdf/265041/trends-in-the-us-uninsured.pdf

70. Lewis, N. A. (2019, February 10). The real reasons women of color lack access to health care. MSN. Retrieved November 1, 2021, from https://www.msn.com/en-us/health/wellness/the-real-reasons-women-of-color-lack-access-to-health-care/ar-BB1enAEX?ocid=msedgntp

71. Frey, W. H. (2018, December 18). Black-White segregation edges downward since 2000, census shows. Brookings. Retrieved November 1, 2021, from https://www.brookings.edu/blog/the-avenue/2018/12/17/black-White-segregation-edges-downward-since-2000-census-shows/

72. Grant, T. (2010, March 9). Study finds median wealth for single black women at $5. Post-Gazette. Retrieved November 1, 2021, from://www.postgazette.com/business/businessnews/2010/03/09/Study-finds-median-wealth-for-single-black-women-at-5/stories/201003090163

73. Melvin, L. (n.d.). Z quotes: Quotes for all occasions. A. Retrieved April 16, 2022, from https://www.azquotes.com/

74. Centers for Disease Control and Prevention. (2019, April 16). About NCHS - NCHS fact sheets - NCHS data on racial and ethnic disparities. Centers for Disease Control and Prevention. Retrieved November 1, 2021, from https://www.cdc.gov/nchs/data/factsheets/factsheet_disparities.htm

75. Trawalter, S. (2020, June 30). Black Americans are systematically under-treated for pain. why? Frank Batten School of Leadership and Public Policy | University of Virginia. Retrieved November 1, 2021, from https://batten.virginia.edu/about/news/black-americans-are-systematically-under-treated-pain-why

76. Cusick, J., (2018, July 9). Health disparities by race and ethnicity. Center for American Progress. Retrieved February 13, 2022, from https://americanprogress.org/article/health-disparities-race-ethnicity/

77. Sokolove Law Team (2020, December 15). Replacing medical errors, covid-19 becomes the 3rd-leading cause of death in the U.S. Sokolove Law. Retrieved November 1, 2021, from https://www.sokolovelaw.com/blog/covid-19-is-3rd-leading-cause-of-death-in-the-u-s/

78. Carrie, A. (2021, March 18). The 8 most common root causes of medical errors. Always Culture. Retrieved November 1, 2021, from https://alwaysculture.com/hcahps/communication-medications/8-most-common-causes-of-medical-errors/

79. Mason, R. J. (2008, August 9). Surgery for appendicitis: Is it necessary? Surgical infections. Retrieved November 1, 2021, from https://pubmed.ncbi.nlm.nih.gov/18687030/

80. Patients whose emergency surgery is delayed are at higher risk of death (2017, July 10). Retrieved November 1, 2021, from https://medicalxpress.com/pdf418872814.pdf

81. Health Insurance Rights & Protections. HealthCare.gov. (n.d.). Retrieved April 16, 2022, from https://www.healthcare.gov/health-care-law-protections/

82. Health insurance rights & protections. (n.d.). HealthCare.Gov; www.healthcare.gov. Retrieved April 16, 2022, from https://www.healthcare.gov/health-care-law-protections/

83. The Joint Commission stands for Racial Justice and equity. The Joint Commission. (n.d.). Retrieved November 1, 2021, from https://www.jointcommission.org/resources/news-and-multimedia/the-joint-commission-stands-for-racial-justice-and-equity/

APPENDIX

Medical Definitions

Colostomy - A colostomy is an operation that creates an opening for the colon, or large intestine, through the abdomen. A colostomy may be temporary or permanent. It is usually done after bowel surgery or injury. Most permanent colostomies are "end colostomies," while many temporary colostomies bring the side of the colon up to an opening in the abdomen. During an end colostomy, the end of the colon is brought through the abdominal wall, where it may be turned under, like a cuff. The edges of the colon are then stitched to the skin of the abdominal wall to form an opening called a stoma. Stool drains from the stoma into a bag or pouch attached to the abdomen. In a temporary "loop colostomy," a hole is cut in the side of the colon and stitched to a corresponding hole in the abdominal wall. This can be more easily reversed later by simply detaching the colon from the abdominal wall and closing the holes to reestablish the flow of stool through the colon. At the hole, a small open end of your ureter or small or large bowel sticks out through your skin. This is called a stoma, and it will look red or pink. It has no nerve endings, so it shouldn't be painful. Your surgeon will connect a pouch, which collects urine or stool, to your stoma. After an ostomy, you will need an ostomy bag to collect the waste that's expelled from your digestive or urinary system. This connects to your stoma so that it's directly emptied without any added effort.

Ostomy bag - Ostomy bag is worn outside the body to collect waste. The bag is easily concealed underneath clothes. If you've had an ostomy, wearing an ostomy bag is important to avoid any leakage from urine, stool, or gas.

PICC line - A peripherally inserted central catheter (PICC) is a small, soft tube that has been placed in a vein in your arm. It is often used when treatment requires medicines or nutrition for weeks or months. At home, you need to take care of your PICC to keep it working. Because a PICC line has a high infection risk, you must take extra care washing your hands and preventing the spread of germs. This sheet will help you remember what to do to care for your PICC at home.

ACKNOWLEDGEMENTS

I actually wrote my first book with illustrations at the tender age of twelve. It was entitled, "The Spell That Never Worked," about a princess who failed to turn a frog into a prince. Although it was never published, I did believe one day, I would become a published author. Upon completing my Ph.D. in Chemical Engineering, my dissertation with the title, "Development of Flouroether Amphiphiles & Their Applications in Heterogeneous Polymerizations in Supercritical Carbon Dioxide," was published in 1997. It was followed by myriad technical papers in both engineering and healthcare journals. Although, my engineering acumen yielded many honors and awards, I was not fulfilled. I had a strong desire, that soon became a mission, to contribute to my community. There are many people who I would like to acknowledge who supported me on this journey despite challenges and other obstacles.

I would like to thank my beloved sister, Diana R. W. Bennett for your endless support and encouragement. I never thought that this book would be possible, but you provided me inspiration, along with much needed wisdom, guidance and personal experiences. My genius nephew, Daniel Ortiz, thank you for listening to my long diatribes and brainstorming ideas about the toolkit. I appreciate your unwavering support. My beautiful niece, Diamond Williams, I greatly appreciated your review and patience while I shared my random thoughts, ideas, and vision without judgment. My publisher, Dr. Sherrie Walton, thank you for believing in me. Your knowledge and experience have impacted my life forever.

I am so very grateful for my husband, Richard Johnson, who reminded me daily that I was valued and my book was well worth the investment of my time, energy, and effort. He is my partner and life coach. I am deeply indebted to my parents who shaped my life. My beautiful and industrious mother who taught me to how to trust in God, and believe that all things are possible. I am truly blessed.

ABOUT THE AUTHOR

Dr. E. J. Johnson is one of eight children born in Pittsburgh, Pennsylvania. She contends that parents must have a vision for their children, and her parents' vision was for all eight children to graduate from college, which they fulfilled. Dr. Johnson exceeded their expectations by obtaining four college degrees; a B.S., M.S., Ph.D. in Chemical Engineering from the University of Pittsburgh, and an MBA from Wilmington University. The daughter of a minister, Dr. Johnson learned early to always keep God at the center of all life's activities.

Dr. Johnson began her career at Westinghouse Electric Corporation based in Pittsburgh, PA in 1983, as a nuclear engineer working on pressurized water reactors. After leaving Westinghouse, Dr. Johnson held several managerial roles at corporations based in South Carolina including Michelin Tire Corporation, and Monsanto Electronic Materials Corporation. In 1993, Dr. Johnson left corporate America and returned to school to obtain her Ph.D. in Chemical Engineering. In 1997, Dr. Johnson made history as the first African American woman to earn a Ph.D. in any engineering discipline at the University of Pittsburgh. In addition, she received the Coull Award, most outstanding Ph.D. candidate, Aristech Award for outstanding research, and became the first National Science Foundation Fellow at her alma mater.

Upon graduating, Dr. Johnson began her engineering research career at Hercules, Inc. based in Wilmington, Delaware. She received several research awards including the coveted Board of Directors New Research Investigator Award. In 2000, she stepped out on faith and launched her own company, Pioneer Training and Consulting, LLC. Her engineering doctorate coupled with her MBA and Lean Six Master Black Belt certification enables her to bring operational efficiency to any organization. Her consulting work in both the pharmaceuticals and hospital systems allows her to see first-hand the racial disparities in both clinical research and healthcare services delivery. She has been instrumental in leading projects that improve clinical outcomes, patient experience, and health equity.

Dr. Johnson is also known for her motivational and inspirational speaking engagements that focus on mental, physical, spiritual, and financial health as well as servant leadership. Dr. Johnson and her husband, Richard Johnson reside in Delaware where they enjoy spending time with family and friends.

CONNECT WITH ME!

There is nothing more important for me as a consultant than to know if I met the needs of my clients. The healthcare industry is complex and it is imperative for you to learn to how it functions to allow proper navigation.

It would be invaluable for me to hear from you. If there is anything that you would like to share including how you currently voice your concerns about your healthcare, please email me or leave a message on my website.

Email: admin@drejjohnson.com
Website: www.drejjohnson.com

Social media:

Facebook	facebook.com/Voice-Your-Concerns-108899905238774
Instagram	instagram.com/concernsvy/
Twitter	twitter.com/your_concerns
Linked In:	linkedin.com/in/dr-e-j-johnson/

Healthcare Consulting inquiries: admin@drejjohnson.com

To book speaking engagements, email: admin@drejjohnson.com

Books available at www.drejjohnson.com and wherever books are sold.

Made in the USA
Monee, IL
04 November 2026

67387168R00134